COVID-19:
Battle for Survival

COVID-19:
Battle for Survival

Prof. Madhu Rajput

KALPAZ

First Published, 2020

Published by

Kalpaz Publications
C-30, Satyawati Nagar,
Delhi – 110052
Ph.: 011-47034999, 9811692060
www.kalpazpublications.com
E-mail: kalpaz@hotmail.com

Printed at: Gyan Press, Delhi

Cataloging in Publication Data—DK
Courtesy: D.K. Agencies (P) Ltd. <docinfo@dkagencies.com>

COVID-19 : battle for survival / [editor], Prof. Madhu Rajput.
pages cm
Contributed articles.
ISBN 9789353242848

1. COVID-19 (Disease)—India. I. Rajput, Madhu, editor.

LCC RA644.C67C68 2020 | DDC 616.2414 23

Contents

Foreword

The United Nations (UN) Millennium Declaration, signed in September 2000, committed world leaders to combat poverty, hunger, disease, illiteracy, environmental degradation, and discrimination against women etc. achieving the same by 2015, as Millennium Development Goals (MDGs). However, as we failed to achieve the MDGs, the then UN Secretary General attributed the lack of progress to 'unmet commitments, inadequate resources, lack of focus and accountability, and insufficient interest in sustainable development' (UN, 2010). Again world population was persuaded to dream in September 2015, when the UN General Assembly adopted the 2030 Agenda for Sustainable Development that included 17 Sustainable Development Goals (SDGs). Building on the principle of "leaving no one behind", the new Agenda emphasizes a holistic approach to achieving sustainable development for all. Out of these 17 SDGs to transform our world, goal no. 3 pertains to Good Health and Well-being. Among its several targets, it also includes the following:

- By 2030, end the epidemics of AIDS, tuberculosis, malaria and neglected tropical diseases and combat hepatitis, water-borne diseases and other communicable diseases.
- Achieve *universal health coverage*, including financial risk protection, *access to quality essential health-care services and access to safe, effective, quality and affordable essential medicines and vaccines for all.*
- Support the research and development of vaccines and medicines for the communicable and non-communicable diseases that primarily affect developing countries, provide

access to affordable essential medicines and vaccines, in accordance with the Doha Declaration on the TRIPS Agreement and Public Health, which affirms the right of developing countries to use to the full the provisions in the Agreement on Trade Related Aspects of Intellectual Property Rights regarding flexibilities to protect public health, and, in particular, provide access to medicines for all.

- Substantially increase health financing and the recruitment, development, training and retention of the health workforce in developing countries, especially in least developed countries and small island developing States.
- Strengthen the capacity of all countries, in particular developing countries, for early warning, risk reduction and management of national and global health risks.

Over last two decades we witnessed three epidemics/pandemics like the SARS (2003) affecting 26 countries, more than 8000 patients and approximately 10% mortality, MERS (2012), 2500 cases with 35% mortality and EVD (Ebola) - A total of *28,616* cases of EVD and *11,310* deaths were reported in Guinea, Liberia, and Sierra Leone. There were an additional 36 cases and 15 deaths that occurred when the outbreak spread outside of these three countries. We all thought and believed that life expectancy has gone up globally due to control over communicable diseases. We were all the time focusing on Epidemic of non-communicable diseases like the diabetes, obesity, hypertension, metabolic syndrome, cardiovascular diseases and related diseases and injury in the new millennium. None of us ever imagined, anticipated, or had any premonition of starting a new year 2020 with something completely off the menu of communicable diseases. Yes, there have been warnings and caution by former US President George Bush long ago and more recently in 2015 by Bill Gates about future wars not being fought with missiles but with microbes, which included both bacteria and virus. We did not believe that these forecasts would become a reality so soon.

We did not realize that Year 2020 will be remembered in history as the gravest existential crisis for human race. It is an unprecedented situation that all of us are facing in the wake of novel corona virus

SARS COV2 causing a disease named by WHO as COVID - 19. The whole world was caught unawares by the disease that has affected millions of people. At the time of writing this foreword on 10th August 2020, number of Coronavirus Cases globally stands at 20,074,993, deaths at 734,888, those recovered 12,931,626. For our country these numbers are 22,42,385 (cases), deaths 44,823, those recovered 15,59,293.

The pandemic has overwhelmed and humbled even the best medical infrastructure in developed countries, which fell short to stop the virus in its trajectory leading to loss of lives. India being an emerging nation with sub-optimal socio-economic-healthcare infrastructure indicators has comparatively done better on the initial containment, recovery rates and deaths (crude mortality). It seems we did get dividend of relatively younger population. Majority of deaths involved elderly patients with co-morbidities, although even younger patients have died. Despite inadequate health infrastructure, the medical community has risen to the challenge to the best of its ability and has been hailed for its service to the humanity by the general populace. Almost 200 doctors have succumbed to COVID-19 contracting the illness in the line of duty. Awareness, precaution and community participation on a larger scale is necessary to minimize the infection in the community and keeping the low mortality rate till the scientists dedicatedly working towards it, are able to find a vaccine. Even in the mid-March 2020, we did not anticipate that this pandemic shall take the shape of today. The role of WHO came under severe criticism due to its inadequate response in cautioning the world community well in time. WHO was all the time seen defending the country of origin of this illness i.e. China. WHO delayed in terming the problem as Public Health Emergency of International Concern (PHEIC) to begin with (30/01/2020) and later inordinate delay in terming the epidemic in WUHAN as Pandemic on 11th March 2020 avoiding any finger pointing at China. WHO believed whatever Data was fed by China, which did not give correct picture of the epidemic in Wuhan.

The edited book titled **"COVID-19: BATTLE FOR SURVIVAL"** by Prof. Madhu Rajput is an exhaustive description and insightful collection of research papers on the impact of this crisis on various aspects of our lives. The first chapter "Pandemics: The Danse Macabre since Ages" by *Colonel Gurusaday Batabyal,* itself impressed me. It traces comprehensive historical dimensions of pandemics from 430 BC into early centuries of first millennium and then in the second millennium. I have found that all the fourteen chapters have uniqueness by inclusion of our ancient wisdom. The book **"COVID-19: BATTLE FOR SURVIVAL" is a must-read book for all sections of society and I am confident that the book will have a large audience and readership (both national and international) because of the depth of knowledge and information it provides.** In the times of death, desperation, deprivation, it is the right approach to take a deeper look at the damage done to socio-economic fabric and psychosocial well-being, with an intention to rebuild and recast the mould of our erstwhile living habits. The book delves into a wide variety of sub-themes related to Covid-19, enriching the knowledge on the subject so intricately related to every human being. The book successfully touches upon various segments of society, economy, polity, giving voice to even those on the periphery. I appreciate the focus of the author towards providing hope and suggestions to tide over the crisis in a united manner, with an endeavor to avoid a recurrence of this sort and holistically move towards a more sustainable and equitable living.

Covid-19 is the trigger for the great awakening, perceiving and utilizing it as an opportunity to reframe our relations with other living beings, while hauling up our governance and infrastructure would be the key to survival and real progress. COVID crisis has also given us opportunity to strengthen our healthcare infrastructure by allocating necessary portion of GDP in federal budget. Pandemic exposed surmountable weaknesses in public sector healthcare infrastructure in the country. There were few positive aspects of lockdown by reducing pollution as suddenly air quality improved significantly in most cities. Also road deaths due to accidents went down during lockdown. However, lockdown brought about tremendous financial misery affecting practically every section of society due to closure of businesses across all sectors (industry, hospitality, travel, transport etc.). It seems economic recovery will take longer than anticipated. Till then, we shall keep reinventing ourselves. Innovation, adaptation and sustained efforts are vital to emerge stronger for the future.

Best wishes!

Dr. M. C. Mishra

Former Director,

All India Institute of Medical Sciences (AIIMS)

New Delhi.

Date:

10th August 2020

Preface

As I write these lines, humanity is undergoing an unprecedented challenge, at least for our generation. The novel Coronavirus which has swept across the world has wreaked havoc and is still continuing its dance of death, with hapless humans running helter-skelter to find a cure to it. The nature and enormity of the pandemic has shaken the collective consciousness of the world and has shattered all the established norms. From socialising to social distancing, globalization to the quest of being self-reliant, the disease has reversed the plan on which human beings had woven their existence till now. In a truly shocking manner, the whole world suddenly went under the lockdown. An invisible virus sent the giant and so-called superior most creature of the planet, who was pompously on the voyage of conquering the land, sea and sky, hiding in their homes. The vacant streets, the eerie quietness, the unseen shadow of the virus lurking everywhere and the overwhelming fear of the unknown, seemed like a scene from a horror movie. Unexpected, unthought of, sudden, and severe that's how the corona virus crept onto us. Its impacts ranged from economy, to environment, to socio-psychological issues to geopolitics. No sphere of life has remained the same as before. The New Normal is here and we have to learn to adjust with it.

The loopholes in health system have been brought to limelight, however the doctors, nursing staff and the cleaning staff have valiantly risen to the challenge. A new team of Corona Warriors has emerged from various quarters, resiliently contributing in the fight against corona virus. The focus however shall be on hauling up the entire health infrastructure, with a renewed drive on prevention which shall encapsulate dedicated research in the field of infectious diseases. In terms of India, it has realized in a hard way a lesson long pending- to strive to be self-reliant in the production of API (Active Pharmaceutical Ingredients) for which it depends heavily on China. Being a leading supplier of generic drugs, India has the potential to emerge as the manufacturing pharmacy of the world, with an additional ingredient of goodwill added as a friend for other nations and has taken initial steps towards it by announcing to launch three bulk drug parks and production-linked incentives for the pharmaceutical companies, which is laudable.

In the field of economy the situation is similar to the 1929 Great Depression where millions have lost their jobs, innumerable people have been thrown below the poverty line and the world economy has contracted. Leisure industries such as travel, tourism, hospitality and fashion have been hit the hardest as people struggle or save to spend on only necessary requirements. The bail out packages to the companies including NBFCs and MSMEs have been launched. India in its bid to revive ground level economy is focusing on SHGs (Self Help Groups) and entrepreneurship. In long term the inward shift may help the domestic industry get a strong foothold inside and outside the country. The orientation shall be to improve the quality and make it competitive in the foreign market, however a distinction will have to be made between self-reliance and protectionism. The changed demography due to reverse migration to villages will have to be taken into consideration when formulating the revival schemes. The crisis has also come along with an opportunity to restructure our economy, and accommodate the aspirations of lower classes into the grand schemes, to utilize India's demographic dividend wisely and harness the potential of digital technology to evolve innovative ways to conduct business while maintaining social distancing norms. The time is ripe to implement some elements of Gandhian economic model of village industries into our economic ecosystem.

Along with survival, human beings need emotional well-being too. By forcing people to remain indoors and by cutting off the emotional support garnered by meeting and talking to friends, the pandemic has put a serious strain on mental health. While the demand of adjusting with the violent disruption in normal life in itself is severe, the economic hardships and closing off the social channels of venting out the stress has increased frustration in people of all age groups, but especially the vulnerable category i.e. children, elderly and the differently abled are struggling to make sense of the situation. The need of the hour is to instill a feeling of connectedness, encourage communication and be empathetic towards the psychological stress people around us are undergoing. Families have got more time to bond but the bonding needs to be now extended to the entire humanity. In the times of crisis, hope and the feeling of being loved are very important tools for survival, hence awareness regarding the importance of mental health and creation of infrastructure for official help needs to be taken up on priority. A collective consciousness of self-belief and the belief in human beings' capability to rebuild their lives should be awakened. Religious leaders, civil society organisations and role models can play a great role in spreading hope, faith, positivity, harmony and creation of an overall resilient mood in the society. The example of His Holiness the Dalai Lama is worthy of emulation here as the leader has been emphasizing on the concept of "One Human Family" to ward off depression, loneliness and sadness in the wake of the pandemic.

Another feature that has come prominently into focus is our relationship with Nature. Prior to the pandemic the way human beings were on a collision course with nature, and the resultant response in terms of climate change, increased number of natural calamities and far reaching consequences staring in our face, and the way during lockdown the environmental indicators drastically improved, with rivers getting cleaner, air getting fresher, and animals roaming without fear has proved that the anthropological actions are the actual culprits behind environmental degradation. It has also highlighted the need for us to rethink our developmental plans, incorporate environment preservation as one of their elements, rather than being the destructive force, and devise sustainable ways to use natural resources. If we do not, it will be at our own peril and we can ill afford that, as the pandemic just showed us. The planet is for all the children of nature, not just human beings and we will have to accommodate them or else the number of infectious zoonotic diseases is going to rise, warn scientists.

Therefore, for the good of all, we need to rescind our superior and marauding attitude and live like one of the components of ecosystem. Technology shall be harnessed fully to create greener buildings, promote solar energy, soil conservation, and biodiversity conservation. Utilising local traditional knowledge and international level collaborations to adopt best practices can be a great start to it, backed by a genuine conviction and drive to mend our ways.

While the origin of the virus has sparked a debate and strong anti-China sentiment prevails in the world, the geo-political equations are being reshaped. The manner in which the information is said to be deliberately withheld and the dealing of WHO of the pandemic has raised suspicions against the nation which has maintained a belligerent attitude, in fact has taken to bullying tactics by flexing its military muscle in its neighbourhood, be it the border stand-off with India, or marine clash with Vietnam, or the new Security Law in Hong Cong. The world is joining up against the rogue nation. India has played its role well as a responsible regional and emerging global power by extending medical help extensively and aiding evacuation of foreign nationals. An attempt to revive SAARC by PM Modi has been well received. India has taken up global roles as the WHO executive Committee Chairperson and winning the UN non-permanent seat. While the world envisions India as the strong antitheses to expansionist and dominating China, India perceives its role as a supporter of democracy, with a shared and transparent vision of peace and prosperity in neighbourhood and beyond. It is time for collaboration with like- minded nations and progress towards enforcing a rule-based, harmonious coexistence.

While in our rebounding phase, we pay attention to all other areas, we shall not forget to look inwards, at the centre of our families, societies and humanity- the women. In past resurgences, be it after the Great depression or the World Wars or a natural calamity, women have been instrumental. They have an amazing capacity to withstand pressure, hold together families and nations, and be a force multiplier in any revival or welfare scheme. By nature, they are the nourishing force, hence acknowledging their contribution and removing barriers from their way to enable full utilization of their potential is imperative and obligatory. The lockdown has brought to fore the ugly patriarchal face of our societies across the world, reflected in the increased figures of domestic violence during the period. They may also be in the firing line on economic front as companies shrink their staff, and therefore the progress done on the front of women autonomy may suffer a setback. However, the examples of resilience, dedication, and leadership set by women across the world in various capacities i.e. doctors, nurses, ASHA workers, women political leaders of Scandinavian countries, psychologists, environment workers, awareness generators, self-help group members keeping up the supply of masks, and sanitisers has enhanced their respect and raised faith in their fighting spirits- be it against the virus or for their rights. Institutional support, societal changes, structural reshaping will go a long way in creating a more egalitarian set up. When in crisis, all the forces shall be combined against the common enemy and hence the prudence dictates that individual nations and the world join hands, transcending barriers of gender, religion, race, caste. Unity is not an option but necessity when it is a question of survival. In the larger interest of humanity also, the divisive lines shall be blurred as far as possible and the force of synergy unleashed for mutual progress.

In the words of an anonymous writer, "Be open to adjustments. There's nothing about this current moment in history that allows for stubbornness". Flexibility, innovation, mindfulness, cooperation, and a will to survive are the weapons to win any battle. It is no doubt a tough time for humanity but it is also an opportunity to introspect and course correct, to emerge as better human beings, to begin with. This book is a compilation of articles highlighting various aspects related to COVID-19 starting from the historical perspective, geopolitical implications, socio-economic and psychological impacts, environment, media coverage and fashion industry, the challenges and ways to overcome them. It is an attempt to vent out our worries, ponder over the solutions and do a collective brain storming to find a better way of life in harmony with each other and nature. We hope for the shedding off of all the negative layers from human heart and actions, and the sparkling of inner luminescence to overcome the darkness. In solidarity with the valiant warriors- against Corona and on the borders, in prayer for the well-being of all across the boundaries!

My heartfelt gratitude to all the contributors who have provided their valuable time and effort in making this work possible. I as an editor have only compiled the articles, and given them a semblance of a book. The views expressed in the articles are of respective authors, and the editor has no role in it.

Prof. Madhu Rajput

Lucknow, 07 July, 2020

List of Contributors

1. Colonel Gurusaday Batabyal, Ph.D., retired Army Officer, Visiting Faculty in various Universities, teaching Modern History of South Asia and International Relations.
2. Dr. Gouri Sankar Nag, Professor of Political Science, Sidho-Kanho-Birsha University, W.B & Coordinator of the Atish Dipankar Srij'nan Centre for South Asian Studies, S-K-B University, W.B., Dr. Manas Mukul Banyopadhyay Associate Professor, PG Department of Pol. Science, Hooghly Mohsin College, W.B & Arpan Bhattacharya, Assistant Professor & Head, Department of Political Science, Ramananda College, Bishnupur, W.B.
3. Squadron Leader Toolika Rani (retd), Research Scholar, Department of History, Babasaheb Bhimrao Ambedkar University, Lucknow.
4. Dr. Shreya Pathak, Assistant Professor, Department of History, Vasanta College for Women, (Admitted to the Privileges of Banaras Hindu University), Varanasi.
5. Prof. Madhu Rajput, Former Head, Department of Western History, Lucknow University, Lucknow.
6. Dr. Shalini Pathak, Guest Faculty, Department of Western History, Lucknow University, Lucknow.
7. Dr. Kumkum Singh, Associate Professor (retd), Former Head, Department of Psychology, RG P.G. College, Meerut.
8. Dr. Subhra Rajput, Associate Professor, Department of English, Dayanand Girls College, Kanpur.

9. Dr. Mani Bansal, Associate Professor, D.A.K. College, Moradabad, Dr. A. K. Agarwal, Associate Professor, T.M.U., Moradabad.
10. Dr. Anantdeep Grewal, Guest Faculty, Northern Indian Institute of Fashion Technology (NIIFT), Mohali, Punjab.
11. Owais Ismaeil, Research Scholar, Department of History, Babasaheb Bhimrao Ambedkar University, Lucknow.
12. Dr. Archna Rathore, Department of English, DAK Degree College, Moradabad.
13. Dr. Achla Sonker, Associate Professor, Department of History, Dayanand Girls (P.G.) College, Kanpur.
14. Colonel Kuldip Singh Grewal (Retd), Formerly Member, Services Selection Board (MoD), President State Ex-Servicemen Welfare Association (SEWA), Punjab.

1

Pandemics: The Danse Macabre Since Ages

— Colonel Gurusaday Batabyal, Ph.D.

Introduction

A rapidly spreading pneumonia of unknown virus detected in Wuhan, China in third week of November 2019 first came to light when defying government orders Dr. Li Wenliang released safety information to other doctors on 30 December 2019. Embarrassed Chinese government officially informed outbreak of this unknown disease to the World Health Organisation (WHO) Country Office in China. A month later the disease was declared a public health emergency of international concern (PHEIC). On 11 February 2020, WHO christened the new coronavirus disease: COVID-19. Dr. Li Wenliang who broke the news first was charged with a crime: sadly he succumbed to COVID-19 four weeks after his disclosure. Due to the severity of the disease and its simultaneous spread across the world affecting large number of people COVID-19 was declared 'pandemic.' Such is the devastating power of this new coronavirus disease that within five months the virus spread to 213 Countries and Territories around the world; WHO as on 01 June 2020 reported globally a total of 6057853 confirmed cases with 371166 deaths.[1] The dreaded disease has so far proved that the world is indeed flat not only because of its geographical reach for its marauding act but more so because it wiped out the distinction between the developed, developing and the underdeveloped countries: north and south were rampaged alike!

But this is not the first time such a disease has brought the world or a country to standstill; history is replete with examples of similar wide-spread diseases. Spread of civilizations and spread of pandemics happened concurrently; pandemics claiming millions of lives since ancient Greece. The ongoing deadly Covid-19 is ever increasing its death tally not to lag too far behind. A few terminologies usually used to denote severity of mass disease need to be explained. WHO site states a disease "outbreak" is the occurrence of disease cases in excess of normal expectancy. Disease outbreaks are usually caused by an infection, transmitted through person-to-person contact, animal-to- person contact, or from the environment or other media. For example, outbreak of cholera in villages in Bengal in nineteenth century. Outbreaks may also occur following exposure to chemicals or to radioactive materials. Occasionally disease outbreaks of unknown aetiology too may occur."[2]

"Epidemic" happens when the disease is affecting or tending to affect a disproportionately large number of individuals within a population, community, or region at the same time. For example typhoid was epidemic.[3] A "pandemic" is an epidemic occurring across the globe, or over a very wide area, crossing international boundaries and usually affecting a large number of people.[4] "By definition, a true pandemic causes a high degree of mortality. By contrast an epidemic affects more than the expected number of cases of disease occurring in a community or region during a given period of time." An "endemic" is present in a community at all times but in low frequency. An endemic is continuous as in the case of malaria in some areas of the world.[5]

Though disease and illnesses have remained inseparable from the humanity since time long past, but earliest histories of illness and disease have not been recorded because of primitiveness and for want of such practice. When the scribes started recording events, they were more interested to record wars and other activities than illness and disease. In 1910, pioneer French Paleopathologists Sir Marcer Arman

Ruffer and A. R. Fergusen examined three mummies of Egypt from the Eighteenth and Twentieth Dynasties(1570-1085 B.C) and found evidence of small pox in the mummified bodies. Most interesting amongst their finding is Ramses V who ruled Egypt and died in 1157

B.C. in his early thirties possibly of small pox which was a scourge in ancient Egypt, China, and India. Shift of demography across the world had been happening since aeons ago; infectious diseases which were transmitted from wild and later from domesticated animals accompanied human beings wherever they shifted. With the increase of humanity's interdependence on one another the scale and spread of these diseases increased manifold, intensified by the communities and traders travelling through land and sea routes. With increased human and animal contact spread of epidemics got accelerated. Plagues, Malaria, tuberculosis, leprosy, influenza, smallpox, and others appeared in the ecosystem since the dawn of civilisation. Advent of medical science notwithstanding, even in this era, outbreaks never ceased to exist though its fury varied.

Pandemics of The Past-Triumph of Death Suspected Typhoid: Ancient Greece, 430 BC

Thucydides recorded the earliest history of pandemic that occurred during the Peloponnesian War in 430 BC. The disease suspected to be a typhoid fever had symptoms of fever, thirst, bloody throat and tongue, red skin and lesions. The pandemic reached Athens when the Spartans laid seize of the walled city after passing through Libya, Ethiopia and Egypt. The city having lost one-third of its population eventually fell to the Spartans. According to Thucydides, Pericles (495- 429 B.C.), a brilliant General, a great statesman and politician "the first citizen" of democratic Athens, succumbed to the deadly disease. The dreaded epidemic typhoid in the walled city of Athens possibly brought an end to the Golden Age of Pericles. Along with it Athenians dominance over the ancient world too came to an end.[6]

The Antonine Plague: 165 to 180 A.D.

This ancient pandemic likely to have originated in China spread westwards through the traders. In 165 CE the deadly disease reached the territory of Roman empire through its troops returning home after campaigning in the Near East who came in contact with the disease during the siege of Seleucia (a major city on the Tigris River in the Near East). During the return journey, Roman army spread the disease northward to Gaul and among troops stationed along the Rhine River. Roman Empire was then at the height of power throughout the Mediterranean world during the reign of Emperor Marcus Aurelius Antoninus (161-180 CE). The pandemic got its name after the emperor. Antonine Plague, sometimes referred to as the Plague of Galen named after the famous Greek physician and author of the great treatise *Methodus Medendi*, who not only witnessed the outbreak but described its symptoms and course in his treatise with adequate details. The outbreak occurred in Rome in two phases, the first phase from 165 to 180 CE affected all of Roman Empire while a second outbreak that occurred in 251-266 CE was no less devastating. More than 2,000 people died daily. Professor Edward Watt writes "Perhaps 10 percent of 75 million people living in the Roman Empire never recovered. Like some beast......the sickness destroyed not just a few people but rampaged across whole cities and destroyed them."[7] Exact cause of this plague remains undetermined, but "based on Galen's description, modern researchers have concluded that the disease affecting the empire was most likely smallpox."[8] Though the Roman Empire survived for the next couple of centuries because of resilience of its people but never recovered from the ruinous blow of Antonine plague that struck the empire; the pandemic is linked to the beginning of its decline and is seen to be as one of the causes for its ultimate fall.

Plague of Justinian

Justinian Plague of 541 CE, world's first great pandemic bubonic plague claiming the lives of millions of people is named after the Roman emperor Justinian I, who reigned The Byzantine Empire between 527-565 CE. In 540 CE the epidemic plague originated in Ethiopia in Africa and spread to Egypt and the Mediterranean. The outbreak in Constantinople was thought to have been carried to the city by infected rats on grain ships arriving from Egypt. Historian John Horgan writes, "The plague arrived in Constantinople (now

Istanbul) capital of Byzantine Empire in 542 CE when Justinian I was in power, almost a year after the disease first made its appearance in the outer provinces of the empire. The outbreak continued to sweep throughout the Mediterranean world for another 225 years, finally disappearing in 750 CE."[9]

The plague, an acute infectious disease caused by the *bacillus Yersinia pestis*, a very pathogenic organism to both humans and animals was discovered many centuries later in 1894 by Alexandre Yersin, a French bacteriologist... symptomatically, initially the infection took the form of large purulent abscesses of lymph nodes, the bubo (L. bubo = 'groin', Gr. boubon = 'swelling in the groin'), this was *bubonic plague*. When bacteraemia followed, it caused haemorrhaging and necrosis of the skin rapidly followed by septicaemic shock and death, due to *septicaemic plague*. If the disease spread to the lungs, it caused an invariably fatal pneumonia, *pneumonic plague*, and in that form plague was directly transmissible from person to person.[10] Genetic studies of modern and ancient Yersinia pestis DNA suggest that the origin of the Justinian plague was in Central Asia and the expansion of nomadic people who moved across the Eurasian steppe, such as the Xiongnu and the later Huns, had a role in spreading plague to West Eurasia from an origin in Central Asia.[11] Plague of Justinian is generally regarded as the first historically recorded pandemic with causal agent as the Yersinia pestis. The pandemic was first reported by The Byzantine historian Procopius in 541 CE from the port of Pelusium, near Suez in Egypt. He was accompanying the Byzantine General Belisarius in Emperor Justinian's wars who witnessed the spread of epidemics. Two other first-hand reports of the plague's ravages were by the Syriac church historians John of Ephesus and Evagrius Scholasticus. "According to Procopius in his History of the Wars, the death toll in Constantinople, when it struck in spring of 542 CE and raged for four months, reached 10,000 a day. Although this figure is probably exaggerated, the plague did profoundly affect the population, both in terms of the victims and the survivors, and as such, was a worthy historical topic for Procopius. After devastating the capital, the plague continued to spread throughout the entire empire, remaining endemic after 542 CE until the middle of the eighth century."[12] In his book "Epidemics and

Society" Frank M. Snowden, Yale University Professor of History of Medicine wrote that "definitive accounts of this plague have largely vanished. However, diaries from Procopius, a noted historian back then, indicate that many thought the end of civilization was upon them."[13]

Justinian plague is estimated to "have killed between 30 and 50 million people, about half the world's population at that time, as it spread across Asia, North Africa, Arabia, and Europe."[14] The plague threatened annihilation of the whole human race. No wonder why many of that era thought of world coming to an end.

Black Death

After the Plague of Justinian (542–546 CE), was The Black Death (1346-53 CE), second pandemic of bubonic plague caused by the bacterium Yersinia Pestis, circulated by rats and fleas. It took a toll of an astronomical figure of almost 200 million people in Eurasia and North Africa. In the human history the devilish plague gets recorded as the "most fatal pandemic and the greatest catastrophe ever". There has been much debate on the origin of the term "Black Death". Describing "death as black" formed part of the ancient phraseology; its use is found in Homeric epic Odyssey to describe the monstrous Scylla, with her mouths "full of black Death.[15] Roman philosopher Seneca the Younger, may have been the first to describe an epidemic as 'black death', (Latin: mors atra) in his magnum opus Odepus but only in reference to the acute lethality and dark prognosis of disease.[16] European languages had different names of this most fatal pandemic like "the great dying" or simply "the plague" but until 1750s the English term "Black Death" to specifically refer this catastrophic plague of 1346-53 CE was not used. In English it was simply known as "the pestilence" or "pestilentia". Though used sparingly, "Bubonic/ pneumonic plague epidemic of 1347-53", a modern name, was introduced in English in 1823 by Elizabeth Penrose's A History of England.[17]

The great plague traces its origin in China and Inner Asia which spread to Euro-Asia mostly through traders and troops mainly by two routes; by land Southwards and by sea across the Black Sea into

Mediterranean Sea. Outbreak of Black Death occurred in the autumn of 1346 when the massive Tartar army under the Mongolian ruler Kipchak Khan Janibeg was besieging the Genoese (Italian) trading port of Kaffa (now Feodosiya) in Crimea. From Kaffa, Italians fled on their ships westward to Mediterranean ports. They were accompanied by an invisible enemy "Black Death".[18] Shipping has much to do with the spread of the disease. "Western crusaders seeking to attack the Holy Land prompted innovations in shipbuilding and these larger and faster ships carried large quantities of goods over extensive trade networks but they also carried the deadly pathogen."[19] Wherever the ships went the traders exchanged goods along with this unseen plague. Through land routes the mighty army of Black Death marched to "Sicily (1347), North Africa, mainland Italy, Spain, and France (1348), and Austria, Hungary, Switzerland, Germany, and the Low Countries (1349). Almost concurrently, another ship from Calais carried the plague to Melcombe Regis, Dorset, in August 1348. After reaching Bristol the disease spread rapidly throughout the southwestern counties of England. London faced its brunt between February and May 1349, followed by East Anglia and Yorkshire during that summer. The Black Death reached the extreme north of England, Scotland, Scandinavia, and the Baltic countries in 1350."[20] Neither Napoleon nor Hitler could succeed in conquering Russia but the great army of Black Death did. It broke through the territory of the city state of Novgorod in the late autumn of 1351 and after a pause during the severe Russian winter army of Black Death conquered Moscow in 1953. After ravaging the historic city of Moscow, the disease also reached the Mongolian border from the west, but mercifully its fury was mellowed down.[21]

One of the primary sources on the outbreak was the Italian writer and poet Giovanni Boccaccio (1313-1375 CE), best known for his work The Decameron; its preface described symptoms of the disease. A few other eye witness writers of that genre also chronicled the catastrophic disease. "Although Boccaccio claims that the first symptom of the disease is the appearance of buboes, most records of the plague indicate that it began with fever, then body aches and fatigue, and then the buboes breaking out on the body."[22] A holistic analysis indicate, all three types of plague- bubonic, pneumonic and septicemic were likely present during Black Death which hit some areas much more severely than others therefore death toll varied from place to place and country to country. Normandy, for example, almost lost whopping 80 percent of its population. Italy was equally competing in this "*danse macabre*". Contemporary Italian writer Agnolo di Tura who lost his wife and five children during this period chronicled his experience from Siena, where the plague arrived in May 1348. An excerpt from his oft quoted overwhelming shock and grief tells it all:

> "Father abandoned child, wife husband, one brother another; for this illness seemed to strike through the breath and sight. And so they died. And none could be found to bury the dead for money or friendship. Members of a household brought their dead to a ditch as best they could, without priest, without divine offices ... great pits were dug and piled deep with the multitude of dead. And they died by the hundreds both day and night ... And as soon as those ditches were filled more were dug ... And I, Agnolo di Tura ... buried my five children with my own hands. And there were also those who were so sparsely covered with earth that the dogs dragged them forth and devoured many bodies throughout the city. There was no one who wept for any death, for all awaited death. And so many died that all believed it was the end of the world". Carmelite friar Jean de Venette in his 14th century French chronicle wrote, "The plague hit hard and fast. People lay ill little more than two or three days and died suddenly….He who was well one day was dead the next and being carried to his grave."[23]

Exact figure of death toll will possibly never be known. With up to two-thirds of sufferers dying from the disease, it is estimated that between 30% and 50% of the population of those places affected died from the Black Death. The pandemic toll finally totalled to an astounding figure up to 200 Millions! "God's Hand Was Unstrung" - existential reflection on life recorded by contemporary Italian historian Matteo Villani. No wonder why bewildered people of that era thought of collapse of civilization!

Smallpox

Smallpox an acute contagious viral disease, with fever and pustules (smallpox sores) that usually leave permanent scars was caused by the Variola virus whose exact origin is not known. Early written descriptions of the disease resembling small pox appeared in China (4th Century), India (7th century) and in Asia Minor (10th century). It gets its name from the Latin word for "spotted" referring to the raised, pustular bumps that break out over the face and body of those affected. Donald Hopkins in his book 'The Great Killer Smallpox' writes, "Smallpox was a scourge in ancient Egypt, China and Greece….First human victims of smallpox probably lived in one of the earliest concentrated agricultural settlements in Asia or Africa sometime about 1,000 B.C."[24] Traces of smallpox pustules were found on the head of Egyptian mummy of the Pharaoh Ramses V who died at the age of forty in 1157 BC is thought to be one of the earliest known victims of the disease.[25] Conquerors, traders and crusaders spread the disease to Asia, Africa, and Europe. During 6th Century smallpox reached Japan through the trading activities between China and Korea. Arabs during their expansion activities in 7th century spread smallpox into northern Africa, Spain, and Portugal. After couple of centuries later during 11th Century Smallpox set its foot in Europe through Crusaders while they were spreading Christianity. During 15th century, smallpox got its access in western Africa through Portuguese colonisation. After Columbus's discovery of a sea route to America in 1492 the dreaded disease eventually reached there during European colonization in the 1500s. In the next two centuries European colonisers and the African slave trade took the smallpox to the Caribbean, Central and South America and later to North America. "Historian and demographer [Noble] David Cook estimates that, in the end, the regions least affected lost 80 percent of their populations, those most affected lost their full populations, and a typical society lost 90 percent of its population. Although we may never know the exact magnitudes of the depopulation, it is estimated that upwards of 80–95 percent of the Native American population was decimated within the first 100-150 years following 1492."[26] Interestingly during colonisation process indigenous people who had no immunity died more because of the disease rather than military conquest and smallpox also came to be known as 'New World smallpox'. During 18th Century smallpox travelled to Australia during exploration by the Great Britain.

Out of the two types of Variola viruses, Variola major was more common with much higher fatality rate vis a vis Variola minor. In addition, 'hemorrhagic' and 'malignant' two other most deadly rarer variants existed that invariably resulted in death. The disease mainly spread either through contacts or through contamination of objects used by the inflicted person or through airborne respiratory droplet secretions.[27] Written descriptions of the disease appeared in India in the 7th century and in Asia Minor in the 10th century. On an average smallpox killed around 30 percent of people who caught it and many of those who survived were left blind, sterile with prominent permanent and at times painful scars and pockmarks on the skin. Variolation (named after the virus) one of the early methods introduced in 10th Century in India (cutaneous technique) and China (inhalation technique) to control the spread of smallpox by a process of grinding up dried smallpox scabs from a smallpox patient and inhaling them or scratching them into an arm of a person who had not had the disease ever before. Centuries later Indian way of variolation method spread to Ottoman Empire (former Asia Minor, present-day Turkey) and North Africa for preventing smallpox. Lady Mary Wortley Montagu, the wife of the British Ambassador in Turkey, learned about variolation during her stay there. Herself a smallpox survivor, in addition to variolating two of her children she became the pioneer to introduce variolation into England.

Trial for vaccination began in 1796 by Edward Jenner (1749–1823), an English doctor. To control this devastating disease, the World Health Organization (WHO) in 1959 initiated a plan to rid the world of smallpox which in the initial years did not progress well for lack of funds and commitments. The Intensified Eradication Programme, began in 1967 with renewed efforts, achieved success through surveillance, detection, investigation and mass vaccination campaigns. A three-year-old girl from Bangladesh Rahima Banu, was the last person in the world to have naturally acquired variola major and Ali Maalin, a hospital cook in Somalia was the last person to have naturally acquired smallpox caused by variola minor. Both made full recovery. Janet Parker who worked at the Birmingham University

Medical School in England got possibly infected via an airborne route, was the last person to die of smallpox on September 11, 1978. Dr. Jenner dreamed that vaccination could annihilate smallpox. His dream came true almost after two centuries when on May 8, 1980, 33rd World Health Assembly officially declared 'the world free of smallpox'- a landmark achievement in medical science dealing with public health.[28] Due to lack of authenticated data there are different views on the estimated death tolls of the history's longest disease. Ramses (1157 BC) is not the only royal who was victim of smallpox; many centuries later six more monarchs Queen Mary II of England (1694), Emperor Joseph I of Austria (1711), King Luis I of Spain (1724), Tsar Peter II of Russia (on 30 January 1730-the very day he got married), Queen Ulrika Elenora of Sweden (1741), King Louis XV of France (1774) and King Louis XV of France (1774) became victim of this dreaded disease. An estimated 300 million people died from smallpox in the 20th century alone according to Colette Flight of BBC and around 500 million people died in the last 100 years of its existence.[29] How rightly Edward Jenner called the virus "speckled monster."

The Cholera Pandemics (1817-1923)

Cholera has ravaged human settlements since time immemorial. Record of the disease is available in the ancient medical books in India, China, Arabia, and Europe chronicled by Greeks and Romans. "The word 'cholera' appeared first in the Hippocratic corpus (460–377 BC) and was referred to as a sporadic diarrheal disease. Galen (129–216 AD) described an illness that is now believed to be cholera"[30]......The disease believably is named by joining two Greek words 'chole' (bile) and 'rein' (to flow); thus meaning the flow of bile. However, in 1622 Alexander Trallianus said that the word has come from 'cholades' which means intestine, as the evacuations were often serous (producing serum) and not bilious. In 1669, English physician Thomas Sydenham (1624-1689), used the term 'cholera morbus' in describing an epidemic in London. The ancient Indian medical texts, Susruta Samhita–mentions a diarrheal disease known as Visucika (Sanskrit name means a disturbance of stomach and intestines generally).[31] It is caused by eating food or drinking water contaminated with a bacterium called Vibrio cholerae. Many infected with this bacterium may not develop any symptoms, amongst those who have symptoms, usually majority are mild cases; only a miniscule percentage develop acute watery diarrhoea with severe dehydration which may become fatal if untreated.

Seven cholera pandemics have occurred in the past 200 years, with the first pandemic originating in Jessore in Bengal (India) in 1817, in addition to recent outbreaks in South America (1990s), Africa (2000s) and Yemen (2010s). Cholera is now endemic in many countries which implies confirmed cholera cases were detected during the last 3 years with evidence of local transmission and not imported from elsewhere Cholera is an easily treatable disease. The majority of people can be treated successfully through prompt administration of oral rehydration solution (ORS). Currently there are three WHO pre- qualified oral cholera vaccines: Dukoral, Shanchol, and Euvichol-Plus. In 2014 the Global Task Force on Cholera Control (GTFCC), with its Secretariat based at WHO, was revitalised. A global strategy on cholera control with a target to reduce cholera deaths by 90% was launched in 2017. A resolution promoting control of cholera and endorsing "Ending Cholera: A global roadmap to 2030" was passed in May 2018 at the 71st World Health Assembly.[32] The WHO estimated that each year there are 1.3 million to 4.0 million cases of cholera, and 21000 to 143000 deaths worldwide due to cholera. "Recently, the re-emergence of cholera has been noted in parallel with the ever- increasing size of vulnerable populations living in unsanitary conditions", the organization said on its website.

The Influenza Pandemic of 1918 - Spanish flu

The influenza virus causes a highly contagious respiratory illness in humans and is an ancient epidemic disease. In 5th century BC Hippocrates described it as "Cough of Perinthus." The influenza pandemic gets traced to "The H1N1 influenza pandemic in 1918-1919" known as "Spanish Flu" or "La Grippe" was a global disaster. It appeared when the World War I was in its final stage. Spain was unfairly connected with the nomenclature of the flu as the deadly disease did not originate in Spain. On the contrary Spain was the only country which honestly reported the deaths. Mostly other countries suffering from this disease suppressed the news of death toll so that it does not demoralise soldiers and citizens in the midst of the Great War. To maintain morale, World War I censors minimized early reports of illness and mortality in Germany, the United Kingdom, France, and the United States. Newspapers were free to report the epidemic's effects in neutral Spain, such as the grave illness of King Alfonso XIII, and these stories created a false impression of Spain as especially hard hit. This gave rise to the name "Spanish" flu. Historical and epidemiological data are inadequate to identify with certainty the pandemic's geographic origin, with varying views as to its location.[33] It spread through the trade routes and shipping lines sweeping North America, Europe, Asia, Africa, Brazil and the South Pacific. Whereas other part of the world witnessed 2-3% deaths, in India the mortality rate was extremely high at around 5%. Later it was found that humid tropical weather helped the deadly virus to spread faster. Usually earlier in similar kind of disease mortality rate amongst young children and elderly people were high, but during this pandemic the pattern of morbidity changed -the flu was most deadly for people aged 20 to 40. Doctors were puzzled and helpless; medicines to deal with this killer disease was unavailable then. The spread was reduced through practicc of isolation and quarantine. Molly Billings, in her article on the topic published in Stanford Education wrote, children would skip rope to the rhyme:[34]

I had a little bird,
Its name was Enza.
I opened the window,
And in-flu-enza.

The H1N1 influenza, a virus which caused the pandemic flu came in two waves, starting in1918 and ending in 1920 lasting for 15 months. As many as 500 million- a third of world population at that time got infected, even Woodrow Wilson, President of the United States was not spared, nor was his eldest daughter Margaret…In April 1919, Woodrow Wilson travelled to the Paris Peace Conference where the "Big Four" (France, the U.S., the United Kingdom, and Italy) met for talks on ending the Great War. Soon after arriving, the President became so ill that the talks were nearly derailed."[35]

Spanish flu killed an estimated 50-100 million people worldwide, according to Jeffrey Taubenberger, MD, PhD, writing for the CDC's Emerging Infectious Diseases journal. This included 675,000 people in the United States. The influenza pandemic has been cited as the most devastating pandemics in recorded world history, it killed more people than the Great War (WW-I).[36] Journal of the American Medical Association on December 28, 1918 noted: "The 1918 has gone, a year momentous as the termination of the most cruel war in the annals of the human race, a year which marked, the end at least for a time, of man's destruction of man; unfortunately a year in which developed a most fatal infectious disease causing the death of hundreds of thousands of human beings." The flu reminds of "The Grim Reaper!"

HIV/AIDS: 1981-present

Human Immunodeficiency Virus (HIV) causes acquired immunity deficiency syndrome (AIDS) which interferes with the body's ability to fight infections. AIDS is one of the deadly diseases in human history that appeared in the last century. Its origin is still a puzzle to the researchers as nothing has been conclusively established though four different theories have been propounded namely, (a) *The Hunter Theory*- The most commonly accepted theory states that Simian Immunodeficiency Virus (SIV) found in chimps became HIV in humans after getting transferred to humans through a process known as zoonosis as a result of chimpanzees being killed and eaten or infected chimp biting the hunter, (b) *The Contaminated Needle Theory*- Preston Marx, a virologist opined that use of single syringe for injecting multiple patients without sterilization transmitted viral particles and further mutation and replication of virus which was passed on from one human to other, (c) *The Colonialism/Heart of Darkness Theory* deliberated by Jim Moore, an American specialist in primate behaviour attributed responsibility to colonisers' inhuman and harsh treatments during the late 19th and early 20th century in French Equatorial Africa and the Belgian Congo where many Africans were forced into labour camps with scarce food and poor facilities creating poor health. SIV possibly infiltrated the labours taking advantage of their weakened immune systems to become HIV. (d) *The Conspiracy Theory* points fingers at CIA and talks of AIDS viruses to be used as biological weapons against homosexuals and Blacks.[37] There are couple of other less discussed theories too.

Possibly no one was alerted about the presence of this virus because of ignorance and isolation within the territory of its origin. In 1981, doctors in the United States identified and reported the first cases of AIDS found in gay men in San Francisco and New York. By end of the year there were 270 reported cases of severe immune deficiency among gay men; 121 of them had died. It was found that besides gays, a drug injected man also got this syndrome. The syndrome was initially called gay-related immune deficiency (or GRID). In September 1982, United States Centres for Disease Control and Prevention (CDC) used the term 'AIDS' (acquired immune deficiency syndrome) for the first time. Same year the disease spread to Haiti and Europe. San Francisco AIDS Foundation (SFAF) in the USA and the Terrence Higgins Trust in the UK were established sensing reach of the disease. In March 1985, the U.S commenced first commercial blood test, ELISA, to detect antibodies to the virus. In September Hollywood heroine Elizabeth Taylor hosted an event in Los Angels and raised more than $1 million for AIDS Project Los Angeles. Two weeks later in October, actor Rock Hudson, a gay became the first high profile fatality of this deadly disease; good hearted actor before his death donated $250,000 to set up the American Foundation for AIDS Research. In later years many celebrities including famous American tennis star Arthur Ashe fell prey to this disease. By the end of 1985, every region in the world had reported at least one case of AIDS, with 20,303 cases in total. The first case of HIV infection as well as first case of AIDS was reported in India in 1986. December 1 is observed as World AIDS day since 1988. By March 1989, AIDS spread its horror in 145 countries and WHO estimated there were up to 400,000 cases worldwide.

Majorly, HIV gets transmitted through exchange of body fluids from unsafe sex, contaminated needles, breast milk, and transmission from an infected mother to her baby during pregnancy and delivery. Alan Whiteside asserts, "HIV is not a contagious disease. It is not contracted by sitting next to a carrier on public transport, as might be the case with influenza, or by eating salad contaminated with bacteria, as with cholera. The cause can be identified."[38] There is no cure for

HIV infection, however the virus can be controlled by administering antiretroviral drugs (ARVs) which prevents further transmission. Various initiatives are in place to control this pandemic by many governments and NGOs. WHO is a cosponsor of the Joint United Nations Programme on AIDS (UNAIDS. In 2016, member states of the United Nations, pledged to end the AIDS epidemic by 2030.

According to Global HIV & AIDS statistics 2019 fact sheet (www.unaids.org), it is revealed that from 1980 to 2018, the disease caused an estimated 32 million deaths worldwide. However, because of better medicine and allied facilities HIV infection has become a manageable chronic health condition bringing hope in the infected people who can now lead long and healthy lives. There were approximately 37.9 million people living with HIV at the end of 2018. But most unfortunately the disease has been stigmatised across the geography traumatizing those who are living with it; they have been deprived economically, ostracized socially and abused mostly. Stigma accentuated sufferings of HIV/AIDS infected persons, and it negated efforts to stem the pandemic. The individuals were shy of and unwilling to undergo HIV testing and further treatment. AIDS created deep social and psychological scars. Women, in particular the widows were the biggest sufferers; here is a poignant poem from them describing their psycho-social perspective:

Silence and shame
prejudices and fear
it's all capsulated in a name
that is always so painful to hear
it is difficult to overcome
challenging to understand
it continues to overwhelm
as we fail to comprehend
that it is no enigma
but simply, something called stigma
that is enormously rife
in this process called life.

—Anonymous HIV- positive Women

Swine Flu (2009-2010)

On 24th April 2009, WHO broke the news that Influenza-like illness in the US and Mexico by Swine Influenza A (H1N1) virus has been reported which never before was detected in 'pigs or humans'. Swine influenza (also called swine flu, hog flu and pig flu) is caused by swine influenza virus (SIV) that usually infects pigs and is endemic in pigs. Present 2009 flu outbreak in humans, known as "swine flu", is due to a new strain of influenza A virus subtype H1N1 that contains genes closely related to swine influenza. In 2009 flu outbreak it was for the first time noticed that pigs can become infected with human influenza viruses. "This virus was originally referred to as swine flu but the WHO decided to rechristen it as 'Influenza A - H1N1 virus' on 30th April 2009 in order to avoid confusion over the danger posed by pigs, especially pork consumption by which the disease is not known to occur and to avoid unnecessary slaughter of pigs."[39] People infected by the swine flu had symptoms similar to human flu like fever, cough, sore throat, body aches, headache, chills and fatigue. Soon the influenza started spreading across all the continents mainly through the international travellers. First case of swine flu was reported in India on 16 May at Hyderabad. On 11 June, World Health Organization (WHO) officially declared that A/H1N1 influenza (swine flu) is a global pandemic. The Government of India along with activation of testing and surveillance facilities screened all people entering India via all the international airports. Pregnant women, children younger than 2 years of age, and people with chronic lung disease were more vulnerable in addition to the people from the disadvantageous groups.

In October 2009, vaccination programs began in the US and Europe, but many healthcare workers were reluctant to have the vaccine, even though it is virtually identical to the seasonal vaccines used in previous years, which have a good safety record. Studies proved that a single dose creates adequate antibodies to protect against the virus within about 10 days after vaccination. Center for Infectious Disease Research and Policy estimated 2009 H1N1 infected 11 to 21 percent of the global population of 6.8 billion at the time or around 700 million to 1.4 billion people. Like previous pandemics death toll reported has wide variations. According to WHO, 18,449 reportedly died during 2009 H1N1 flu pandemic but CDC estimated about 284,000 (range from 150,000 to 575,000) death. On 10 August 2010, WHO announced that the H1N1 influenza virus is no more pandemic as it has moved into the post-pandemic period; but cautioned that localized outbreaks of various magnitudes are likely to continue which came true.[40] The Flu has been reappearing occasionally in many countries since it reached the non-pandemic phase. For example, India reported 20,164 cases with 164 deaths as on 24 March 2010 but after remaining fairly dormant for some years in 2015 the instances of swine flu substantially increased to five year highs with over 10,000 cases reported and 660 deaths. Rajasthan, Gujarat, Madhya Pradesh, Maharashtra, Delhi, and Telangana had the highest number of cases and deaths.[41]

Nexus between Pandemics and War

"*Veer Bhogya Vasundhara*"[42] translated into English would read, "The Brave Shall Inherit the Earth", and has remained true since thousands of years. Throughout the history, war has been pursued for many reasons: expansion or protection of kingdom/ state, politico-economic gains and last but not the least struggle for power. History is full of examples how pandemics and epidemics have altered outcome of war along with the fate of the warring empire/state. Thucydides gives details in his seminal work Peloponnesian War (430 BC) how pandemic plague reached Athens from Egypt. He also records that Pericles, a brilliant General and Head of Athens succumbed to the deadly disease in addition to one third of its population including many soldiers and seamen. Pandemic typhoid took a heavy toll of country's economy, administration and most importantly its military. Military became weak- there were hardly any able-bodied men who could be recruited to replace the dead soldiers. The pandemic led to the downwards journey of Athens which in due course changed the Athenians dominance over the ancient world. Historian Dio Cassio records that in 178 AD Roman Republic was paralyzed due to onslaught of smallpox that reached the empire along with the victorious Roman army of General Lucius Verus returning from Syria after defeating the Perthians in the gulf. The deadly Antonine Plague "decimated 90% of the Roman Army, and shrank the labor forces which probably led to the eventual decline of the great Roman Empire."[43]

Procopius chronicled how Justinian Plague collapsed Byzantine Empire because defence and economy collapsed due to innumerable deaths. In 568 CE, the Lombards successfully invaded northern Italy and defeated the Byzantine garrison and fractured Italy; in North Africa and the Near East, encroachment of Arabs could not be stemmed because Byzantine army was so reduced that it became incapable to defend the empire. The decrease in the population due to pandemic deaths had a telling effect on military, economy and administration; the empire began to collapse. Even a smaller scale Ethiopian seize of Mecca (568 AD) failed because of smallpox epidemic. In 1347 AD, the Golden Horde under Jani Beg could not hold the seize in Kaffa (Cremean peninsula) more than four years because the plague reduced their strength to further resist reinforcements from Italy. Both sides withdrew to escape from the plague infected port city and spread the plague during their journey which ravaged many countries. During the period of Black Death, England and France had no choice but to halt the war by calling a truce because both were so weakened by the plague that their combat power reduced drastically.

In 1503 a cholera or suspected pox like epidemic took toll of 2000 men in the army of sovereign Calicut during Vasco da Gama's naval campaign, chronicles Gasper Correa, a Portuguese explorer. In the 16th Century European expansion and colonization in the New World got expedited because the natives with no immunity suffered estimated 20 million casualties due to smallpox pandemic. During the Russian Campaign, Napoleon got defeated because of many reasons like severe winter, lice infected soldiers living in unhygienic conditions etc. But it is important to note that out of his 6 lakh army, 80,000 died of typhus epidemic alone in Lithuania![44] American Civil War got prolonged by two years because of pneumonia and typhoid epidemics. Approximately 660,000 soldiers died (2/3rd strength) due to uncontrolled infectious diseases. Several major operations had to be halted due to epidemics prolonging the operation.[45]

In 1870 during the Franco-Prussian war in Europe, the French army lost 23,400 soldiers to the typhoid epidemic, on the contrary Germans army lost only 278 soldiers because they were vaccinated before the war. During WW-I Spanish flu of 1918 took heavy toll on the American army. It lost more personnel to disease (63,114) than to combat (53,402).[46]

Pandemics and epidemics proved more lethal than most effective weapons which altered outcome of war and destiny of a nation or empire. Ships and soldiers historically had been biggest carriers of contagious plagues and other diseases not only to the war zone but also to their respective countries during their return journey in addition to spreading the pandemics to countries falling enroute their destination. Destructive powers of pandemics gave idea to the war makers to use biological weapons against enemy since many centuries. Possibly it started from Jani Beg, the Mongol General who catapulted plague infected corps of dead soldiers for spreading the disease to weaken his enemy Genoese.[47] Later Genoese fled from Kaffa to Genoa, introducing the Black Death into Europe in 1347. During colonisation in 1763, British distributed blankets from smallpox patients to Native Americans to get them infected. In 1863, Confederates sold clothing from yellow fever and smallpox patients to Union troops, USA. "In the summer of 1864, Dr. Luke P. Blackburn, a Kentucky-born physician turned Confederate agent, allegedly instituted a bioterrorism plot against President Abraham Lincoln…. The plot was unsuccessful."[48] These are just a select few examples; there are many more instances of how the disease virus/bacteria was converted and used as biological weapons since many centuries. International body through multilateral disarmament treaty have banned the entire category of such weapons of mass destruction, which came into force on 26 March 1975.

Gods, Superstitions and Prejudices in the Time of Pandemics

Theurgical beliefs were upheld in ancient civilizations such as India and Egypt. They were of the view that pestilences were unleashed on mankind as punishment for their incorrect behaviour. When Christian era began same concept was further enlarged with belief that God could employ the disease to cleanse men of his sins. In ancient time therefore scourge of pandemics was seen as wrath of or act of God. "Homer wrote in The Iliad of the god Apollo raining plague down on the Greek army with his arrows during the Trojan War, killing animals first, then soldiers. Apollo's arrows came to symbolize disease and death."[49] One of the oldest recorded superstitions about the Bubonic Plague is there in the Old Testament in the story of the Philistines who stole the Ark of the Covenant from the Israelites and succumbed to "swellings."[50]

During The Black Death, instead of fleas and rats as carriers, many pundits mooted the idea of "noxious vapors" or bad air as a breeding ground for pestilence. In religious lines many Christians viewed it "a punishment from God for humanity's sins but could also be caused by 'bad air', witchcraft and sorcery" whereas large number of Muslims believed, "The plague was a merciful gift from God which provided martyrdom for the faithful whose souls were instantly transported to paradise"[51] In 1348, on an inquiry from King Philip VI of France on the causes of the bubonic plague, Professors of medicine of University of Paris in their report ascribed the disease to configuration of stars. As per their report the epidemic occurred because in 1345, three planets [Saturn, Mars and Jupiter] in Aquarius appeared in conjunction, it also coincided with a lunar eclipse around the same time.

All through the history, bias and superstitions thrived during epidemics/pandemics. Italy between 1493 and 1785, restricted movements of Romas; longest persecutions faced through promulgations of innumerable laws "driven partly by the prejudiced view that the Roma people (Romani Gypsies) caused and spread epidemics." In medieval Europe, even Bard of Avon- Shakespeare thought plague and malaria were an atmospheric thing caused by the sun steaming up swamp "vapours."[52] He wrote:

All the infections that the sun sucks up
From bogs, fens, flats, on Prosper fall and make him
By inch-meal a disease!

—Shakespeare's "The Tempest"

The miasma theory of disease originated in the Middle Ages and persisted for centuries. During the Great Plague of 1665, doctors wore masks filled with sweet-smelling flowers to keep out the miasmas poisonous gas.[53]

One of the saddest stories of bias was the case of Mary Malon, an Irish cook who worked in a wealthy residencies in New York Long Island. In early 1900s. Not only she was suspected as the spreader of a mysterious disease typhoid that occurred that time, even she was disgraced by naming the disease after her calling it 'Typhoid Mary'. Poor Mary Malon, without any conclusive proof was "quarantined for 26 years, next to the Riverside Hospital on North Brother Island, where she finally died in 1938. An impassioned exoneration came 63 years later."[54]

Probably the most obnoxious superstitions in modern age are connected with AIDS. Many people still believe the myth that sex with a virgin or young girl can cure men of HIV/AIDS in some part of Africa. "Virgin cleansing" as a therapeutic response to HIV/AIDS is prevalent amongst the Zulu. In Botswana, where nearly 40 percent of the adult population has the virus, this myth is particularly widespread, and some men deliberately seek out young girls for intercourse as a way of avoiding HIV infection. According to Sarawak AIDS Network, or SAN in Malaysia, "prostitute and their customers shake up a can of coca cola and spray their genitals before sex." The belief is that the bubbles in the soda will kill the virus." Bizarre theories from the fertile human brains!

Naming a pandemic or epidemic many a times had geographical orientation in addition to colonial bias. Like Indian Cholera, Asiatic Cholera, Spanish Flu and many such. In 2015, the World Health Organization issued new guidelines for naming new infectious diseases in humans. The guidelines are meant to "minimize unnecessary negative effects on nations.

It is human nature that God is remembered more at the time of danger. Since antiquity, the maxim has been truly followed by many cultures across geographies and religions. Gods and Goddesses were prayed to cure epidemics and widespread illness. Romanians worshipped Febris-god of fever and malaria. Greeks worshipped Apollo -god of healing, medicine, and diseases, and Panacea -daughter of Asclepius who could heal any disease. Besides, Greek mythology talks of Nosoi- spirits of pestilence and disease. Aztec had Chalchiuhtotolin who cured diseases. Babylon too had a plague God named Erra. Irish mythology talks about Brigid- worshipped for her healing power. A Chinese folk lore talks of Tian Hua Niang Ning and believes that the children should worship her for getting cure from smallpox in addition to Wen Shen a deity to cure plague like disease. In Bengal (India) Ola Bibi was worshipped for cholera and Shitala Devi is worshipped in Bengal, North India and Gujrat for pox like disease. The list goes on for such cultural narratives. David Tacey while introducing his book, 'Gods and Diseases' says, "Spiritual forces aren't otherworldly or spooky things - they're the deeper emotional and psychological currents of this world." The connect with God deepens during heightened fear of death. If not divine cure which many would argue against being unscientific, this connect reduces depression, mental stress and anguish.[55]

Conclusion

Traversing through the memory lane of deadly diseases the world has encountered, it gets established that apocalyptic outbreaks of diseases have been occurring intermittently since time immemorial. Mankind let its imagination run wild to find origination of pandemic or epidemic disease; it ranged from wrath of God to wrong constellation of stars; from foul-air to despised people. It is only after the discovery of germ theory, explanation about the mass disease has much changed following a logical scientific reasoning, though superstitions and bias are still prevalent albeit in lesser degree. Introduction of penicillin and other antibiotics supported by vaccination campaigns have resulted in gradual reduction in the death rate. A pandemic like COVID-19 puts heavy pressure on the existing healthcare systems which almost in every country was found inadequate to cope up initially: the speed in which it spread and exponential growth taken all by surprise. Even the developed countries like Italy, USA, UK, and France were helpless. However, efforts were made to cope up and rise to the occasion. On war footing respirators, ventilators, and protective gears were made to meet the increased demand. Many companies like General Motors, Maruti, Mahindra and Mahindra, DRDO changed their assembly lines to produce ventilators to cope with the unprecedented demands.

Restrictions on movement by disallowing or curtailing travels - inland and worldwide though help in slowing the spread of the disease but have a huge socio-economic impact. The world is restless, depressed and economically suffering a lot because of job cuts, business loss, while government revenue is hitting the bottom. Till a vaccine is found and is available in the market, life may not be same again. Governments across geographies are cooperating with others to support research initiatives on finding a vaccine. India has been in the forefront to extend support to many countries with supply of medicines like Hydroxychloroquine tablets and creating a fund for the SAARC countries in addition to pledging support to UK led vaccine research programme. India has also pledged support to BIMSTEC in this hour of crisis. Prime Minister Modi was few notches ahead in the global health diplomacy. Despite all the efforts and sincerity of purpose, securing equitable health care is a difficult job. All affected persons in the underdeveloped or developing world may not get vaccination because of the monetary constraints.

"Health workers and caregivers are inevitably on the front line in a pandemic. While they have an ethical obligation to provide safe care, they do so with the knowledge that they bear a high personal risk of infection."[56] Quarantine is an effective method practiced since many centuries to check spread of the contagion. Venice put this into practice in 14th century in order to keep plague out; ships were not permitted to enter dock for 40 days.[57] Self-discipline, social harmony and community support in response to pandemic have to be the order of the day to live for another good day.

Concealment of epidemics has been oft repeated in the past; an apt example is Spanish flu -1918. Some countries have accused China for hiding the facts about Corona virus attack which led to spread of the disease to many parts of the world through unrestricted travels. WHO has been blamed for failing to play its role in alerting the world timely; suspicion has been raised on WHO's dalliance with China. The media, Facebook, Whatsapp et all have the power both to inform and to misinform. Politically motivated false and negative information doing round have a psychological impact and adding fuel to the fire.

Michigan University Professor of History of Medicine Dr. Howard Markel, drawing lessons from Albert Camus', The Plague, talks of "Four Acts Model" of an Epidemic. During the first act, "progressive revelation," a country or a community slowly acknowledges presence of the killer disease and reveals data on numbers affected and deaths. During Act-II, "managing randomness," when society creates an intellectual framework to understand the erratic behaviour of the disease. Here existing belief system of society including religion's influence is to form part of the narrative. In the next phase, Act-III, "negotiating public response"- is a crucial phase where leadership and those managing the scourge have a tough job in handling, communicating and convincing its citizenry. If not managed and balanced properly the country can lapse into socio-economic turmoil, chaos and in worst case anarchy. Opposition parties in a democracy have to play a positive role and major decisions should be taken after reaching a consensus. The last stage i.e. Act IV, "subsidence and retrospection," is the most vexed act according to Howard Michael because usually complacency starts setting when the epidemic is in its withdrawal phase. Society remains confused for some time because the epidemic goes not with a "bang but with a whimper". The Professor feels that this "four-act model of epidemics is an excellent starting point for our contemplation of pandemics."[58]

Ongoing rampage of Covid-19 is not the first pandemic the world is experiencing and it may not be the last pandemic that would have visited the world. Only posterity will tell if Covid -19 had had that distinction. Medical science despite its progress is unlikely to ever offer full protection from future pandemics because of the antigenic shift where a recognizable virus having undergone an abrupt change surfaces as a different kind of disease. Like, Corona virus is not similar to H1N1 virus; therefore with dissimilar virus, there will be a new challenge to control and cure. This cat and mouse game will continue.

Except for Antarctica, COVID-19 has reached all the continents. International organizations around the world, such as the WHO and the Centres for Disease Control and Prevention (CDC) are monitoring the behaviour and movement of Corona virus. Their findings help health authorities develop strategies for controlling the spread and impact of Covid-19. Ministry of Health, Government of India has thus far played its role well to coordinate, monitor and update all about the disease. Prime Minister Mr. Modi's proactive stance in ensuring lockdown to stem spread of the disease in close co-operations with the state governments had checked spread of virus not to reach exponential stage *ab intio*. Issues like management of migrant labourers, their transportation back home, many unfortunate deaths during their return journey home and miseries undergone are some of the unexpected fall outs during this grim period. But on the positive side many organisations and individuals rendered much help to the needy though need outstripped resources because of humungous number and lack of coordination. Two aspects became very clear; a country like India with such large population needs to enhance its medical infrastructure manifold. Though much has happened from zero start like testing facilities to production of masks and ventilators including constant effort to find a vaccine, much more is needed to be done and most importantly lessons should not be forgotten once the danger is over. How a country or people behave during epidemic has been well captured by Camus in his four act play 'Plague' and much lessons as enunciated before can be learned to take corrective measures. While on health management, one couldn't agree more with Modiji on aspect of "*atma-nirbharta*" (self reliance); the crisis can only be handled then. It is a naked truth that no government or administration in India ever planned or had any credible data on migrant labours. "They were not in anyone's imagination and scheme of things". After this painful episode, Prime Minister and a few Chief Ministers like Yogi Adityanath, Capt. Amrinder Singh have already swung into action to collate data for better management in future. It is felt that a national data bank with real time updates will be needed and that's a huge job. Pandemics have shaped history in many different ways since antiquity. Long sequestering at home as a safety measure, prolonged social distancing and loosing job and loosing kith and kin affect human psychology. Even when the disease reaches endemic stage, anxiety of recurrence and traumatic stress disorders will remain till time heals. Covid-19 bared the truth that "anyone might become ill, anyone might provide comfort". It echoes what Nancy K Bristow said in context of 1918 Flu Pandemic, "Mankind lives on eternal hope". Modern medicine and multi-prong concerted actions besides human resilience, grit and determination will overcome the pandemic in near future. Charlie Chaplin who made all of us laugh said, "Nothing is permanent in this wicked world, not even our troubles". Covid-19 too shall pass.

Let's pray Vedic Peace Chants from Brihadaranyaka Upanishad seeking good health and peace for all:

Om Sarve Bhavantu Sukhinah, Sarve Santu Nir-Aamayaah |
Sarve Bhadraanni Pashyantu, Maa Kashcid-Duhkha-Bhaag-Bhavet |
Om Shaantih Shaantih Shaantih |

English translation of the above prayer originally written in Sanskrit would be:

May everyone be happy, may everyone be free from all diseases
May everyone see goodness and auspiciousness in everything,
May none be unhappy or distressed.
Om peace, peace, peace!

Notes & References

1. WHO covid-19-sitrep report dated 01 June 2020.
2. https://www.who.int/environmental_health_emergencies/disease_outbreaks/ en/ viewed on 16 May 2020.
3. https://www.merriam-webster.com/dictionary/epidemic viewed on 17 May 2020.
4. Last JM, editor. A dictionary of epidemiology, 4th edition. New York: Oxford University Press; 2001.
5. The word "pandemic" comes from the 17th century Greek word "pan-", meaning "all" + "demos," meaning "people or population" = "pandemos" = "all the people." A pandemic affects all or nearly all of the people. By contrast, "epi-" means "upon." An epidemic is visited upon the people. And "en-" means "in." An endemic is in the people. William C. Shiel Jr., MD, FACP, FACR, *Medical Definition of Pandemic*, https://www.medicinenet.com/script/main/art.asp?articlekey=4751, viewed on 18 May 2020.
6. A.W. Gomme, *An Historical Commentary on Thucydides*, II, 145–62.

7. Edward Watt, What Rome Learned From the Deadly Antonine Plague of 165 A.D. SMITHSONIANMAG.COM, April 28, 2020.

8. John Horgan, Antonine Plague, Ancient History Encyclopedia, published on 02 May 2019. https://www.ancient.eu/Antonine_Plague/ viewed on 21 May 2020.

9. John Horgan, Justinian's Plague (541-542 CE), Ancient History Encyclopedia, published on 26 December 2014, viewed in https://www.ancient.eu/article/782/justinians-plague-541-542-ce/ on22 May 2020.

10. John Frith, in History, *The History of Plague – Part 1*. Volume 20 No. 2. https://jmvh.org/article/the-history-of-plague-part-1-the-three-great-pandemics/ viewed on 22 May 2020.

11. Damgaard, Peter de B.; et al. (May 9, 2018). "137 ancient human genomes from across the Eurasian steppes". Nature. 557 (7705): 369–374 quoted in Wikipedia, viewed in https://en.wikipedia.org/wiki/Plague_of_Justinian#cite_note-Damgaard-12 dated 22 May 2020.

12. Michael S. Rosenwald, History's deadliest pandemics, from ancient Rome to modern America, Washington Post, April 16, 2020.

13. Snowden quoted in History's deadliest pandemics, The Washington Post Apr 20, 2020.

14. Ker Than, NATIONAL GEOGRAPHIC, published on January 31, 2014. Viewed in https://www.nationalgeographic.com/news/2014/1/140129-justinian-plague-black-death-bacteria-bubonic-pandemic/ on 22 May, 2020.

15. Homer, Odyssey, XII, 92.

16. Seneca, Oedipus, 164-170. https://en.wikipedia.org/wiki/Black_Death viewed on 23 May 2020.

17. https://www.etymonline.com/word/black%20death viewed on 24 May 2020.

18. Ole Benedictow, Black Death-Greatest Catastrophe, Published in History Today, Volume 55, Issue 3, March 2005 (https://www.historytoday.com/archive/black-death-greatest-catastrophe-ever retrieved on 20 May 2020.

19. Khan Academy article on the Black Death, https://www.khanacademy.org/humanities/renaissance-reformation/late-gothic-italy/beginners-guide-late-gothic/a/the-black-death, viewed on 22 May 2020.

20. https://www.historytoday.com/archive/black-death-greatest-catastrophe-ever & Raza Mohsin, Deadly disease: Epidemics throughout History, https://m.facebook.com/story.php?story_fbid=10158251960089756&id=141343544755&__tn_=-R viewed on 27 May 2020.

21. https://www.britannica.com/event/Black-Death/Cause-and-outbreak. https://www.britannica.com/event/Black-Death accessed on 27 May 2020.

22. Joshua J. Mark, Boccaccio on the Black Death: Text & Commentary, On line Ancient History Enclyopedia published on 03 April 2020.

23. Agnola de Tura, Cronaca Senese 1348 quoted in Negru Catalin, A History of the Apocalypse, (2nd Ed), 2018 Lulu Press, North Carolina, p.133.

24. Donald R. Hopkins, *The Greatest Killer Smallpox*, The University of Chicago press, Chicago (1983), pp. 9-13.
25. Donald R Hopkins, Ramses V-Earliest Known Victim, accessed in WH_1980_May_p.22-26_eng.pdf on 06 June 2020. All researchers agree Pharao Ramses V died young; but his exact age at the time of death has had different views.
26. Michael S. Rosenwald, History's Deadliest Pandemics from Ancient Rome to Modern America, The Washington Post, April 16, 2020.
27. NATIONAL GEOGRAPHIC, https://www.nationalgeographic.com/science/health-and-human-body/human-diseases/smallpox/ viewed on 24 May 2020.
28. "History of Smallpox". Centre for Disease Control, retrieved on 24 May 2020, https://www.cdc.gov/smallpox/history/history.html.
29. Henderson D (2009). Smallpox: the death of a disease. Prometheus Books, New York, p. 12.
30. Sen, Srabani, Indian Cholera: A Myth, Indian Journal of History of Science, 47.3(2012) 345-376.
31. *Ibid.*
32. WHO SITE on CHOLERA updated on 17 January 2019https://www.who.int/news-room/fact-sheets/detail/cholera
33. History of Spanish flu, https://en.wikipedia.org/wiki/Spanish_flu accessed on 21 May 2020. This has been also quoted by many other writers on the topic.
34. Molly Billings, June, 1997 modified RDS February, 2005, https://virus.stanford.edu/uda/ accessed on 02 June 2020.
35. The Influenza Pandemic of 1918, https://virus.stanford.edu/uda/ accessed on 31 May 2020.
36. What 1918 Spanish Flu Death Toll Tells Us About COVID-19 Coronavirus Pandemic, https://www.medicinenet.com/script/main/art.asp?articlekey=228841 accessed on 08 June 2020.
37. Origin and Diffusion of HIV/AIDS,https://shodhganga.inflibnet.ac.in/bitstream/10603/169788/8/08_chapter%202.pdf viewed on 30 May 2020
38. Alan Whiteside (2008), MV/AIDS - A Very Short Introduction', Oxford University Press, USA. http://hdl.handle.net/10603/126970 and http://shodhganga.inflibnet.ac.in:8080/jspui/handle/10603/126970
39. Milind Y Nadkar, Shobha Subramanian, Nayana Ingole, H1N1 Influenza: An Update viewed in https://japi.org/june_2009/07_UA_Swine_Flu.pdf. 39>
40. https://www.cdc.gov/flu/pandemic-resources/2009-h1n1-pandemic.html & WHO Report- https://www.who.int/csr/disease/swineflu/en/ on 22 May 2020.
41. Milind Y Nadkar, Shobha Subramanian, Nayana Ingole, H1N1 Influenza: An Update; viewed in https://japi.org/june_2009/07_UA_Swine_Flu.pdf. 39> on 24 May 2020.
42. Kata Upanishad (Chapter 2, Canto 2, Verse 1).

43. Fears JR. The plague under Marcus Aurelius and the decline and fall of the Roman Empire. Infect Dis Clin North Am 2004; 18: 65-77.
44. Burky T, The Illustrious Dead: The Terrifying Story of How Typhus killed Napoleon Greatest Army, Lanclet Infect Dis 2010; 10:748.
45. J S Sartin, Infectious Diseases During the Civil War: The Triumph of the "Third Army", Clin Infect Dis. 1993 Apr;16(4):580-4. doi: 10.1093/clind/16.4.580.
46. Carol R. Byerly, War Losses (USA), https://encyclopedia.1914-1918-online.net/article/war_losses_usa viewed on 4th June 2020.
47. Roy K, Ray S. War and epidemics: A chronicle of infectious diseases. J Mar Med Soc 2018; 20:50-4.
48. Mathew W. Lively Blackburn, Luke P, Yellow Fever Plot of 1864 Targeted Lincoln, U.S. Cities, July 13, 2014. https://www.civilwarprofiles.com/yellow-fever-plot-of-1864-targeted-lincoln-u-s-cities/. Accessed on 25 May 2020.
49. https://www.history.com/news/how-infectious-diseases-spread-myth-superstition-theories viewed on June 5, 2020.
50. Windy Orent, American anthropologist is quoted in John Horgan, Justinian's Plague (541-542 CE), Ancient History Encyclopedia, published on 26 December 2014.
51. Joshua J. Mark, Black Death, published on 16 April 2020, viewed in https://www.ancient.eu/article/1541/religious-responses-to-the-black-death/ on June 5, 2020.
52. Viewed in quarter.https://www.history.com/news/how-infectious-diseases-spread-myth-superstition-theories. Accessed on 04 June, 2020.
53. Misama Theory, https://www.medicinenet.com/script/main/art.asp?articlekey=19304, viewed on 06 June, 2020.
54. Acharya, Amitangshu, Pandemics and prejudice: When there is an epidemic, social prejudices resurface, The Hindu, 03, 2020. Roma of Europe faced similar persecution. Giorgio Viaggio, in his book Storia Degli Zingari in Italia (1997), has documented 121 laws framed to impose restrictions.
55. Tacey, David, Gods and Diseases, Routledge, London, 2011.
56. Ethical and Legal Considerations in Mitigating Pandemics Disease, Institute of Medicine of the National Academes, Washington, p. 34.
57. https://www.ncbi.nlm.nih.gov/books/NBK54171/ viewed on 2 June, 2020.
58. https://www.ncbi.nlm.nih.gov/books/NBK54171/, accessed on 4 June, 2020.

2

Re-reading 'Arthashastra' During the Current Pandemic: India's Geo-political Concerns and Quest for Astute Neighbourhood Diplomacy

— *Dr. Gouri Sankar Nag,*
Dr. Manas Mukul Banyopadhyay &
Arpan Bhattacharya

Today when almost all members of India's strategic community are virtually perturbed by China's border incursion and bellicosity at Ladakh which is not only startling given India's bold outreach at Doklam in 2017 where a 73 days long stand-off was enough to push back China, but which is also embarrassing in the context of the current pandemic, we find it intellectually gratifying and stimulating to take recourse to Kautilya's Arthashastra in our quest for inputs to devise the lexicon of India's adroit response to her immediate neighbours. The Arthashastra is an ancient Indian Sanskrit treatise inter alia on statecraft, economic policy and military strategy. The more we plumb the depth of the text the more we get awe-struck by the sheer insight with which Kautilya, also identified as Vishnugupta or Chanakya, the chancellor and mentor of the emperor Chandragupta Maurya, dealt with problems in politics including diplomatic suggestions based on hypotheses that he had offered. Though written about 2400 years ago, Kautilya's Arthashastra is a rich reservoir of astute guidance to rulers which is eternal in nature, hence revisiting that thought seems potentially enlightening for our strategic perspective to solve many of India's current military, diplomatic and other imbroglio and predicaments. This acts as a veritable springboard behind our endeavour to rediscover the hidden guidelines embedded in the ancient text in the wake of the Covid-19 pandemic when geo-political threats emerging from the cauldron of India's immediate neighbourhood intensify the gravity of the overall challenge.

In the third century B.C., lived Kautilya, one of the most fascinating characters in Indian history. His seminal work, Arthashastra, ought to be read by all, be they statesmen, or academic scholars. Arthashastra written by Kautilya/ Chanakya/ Vishnugupta (different names of same person) is eloquently referred to for upholding a prodigious formula of '*Saam, Daam, Danda* and *Bhed'* (persuasion, temptation, punishment, and division) as various, different and sequential means to achieve an end. Actually he focused extensively on the conduct of foreign policy, diplomacy and war. One of his popular theories is *Saptanga* theory which preached that the King is the linchpin of the institution of the state, the very basis of the '*Saptanga* organism. "In trying to understand Kautilya's analysis, we have to keep in mind the fact that it is essentially theoretical. Since, in the Kautilyan view, the King encapsulates all the constituents of a state…what Kautilya calls the 'interest of the king' would nowadays be termed 'national interest'…" (L. N. Rangarajan, Koutilya The Arthashastra, Penguine Books, 1992)

In Kautilya's contemporary India there were many small and big kingdoms, not all, however, were monarchical. At the same time, Alexander's invasion of India took place in 326 BC. This incident led to the formation of economic and other kind of ties with some of the countries outside India. There is a discussion in Arthashastra about various alliances to counter the powerful enemy, comparative estimate of power of the allies, entering agreement with renegades, different forms of battle of which Kautilya preferred open fight to pulverize the enemy. Of course, he was astute enough to endorse the dual policy of war and peace although in ancient India, wars between kings were considered normal. Kautilya has discussed in Arthashastra about the duties of such a king who is wishing to be a conqueror, "an ambitious king (known as '*Vijigisu*') who wishes to carve an empire for himself (Basak, 1967). He instructed the '*Vijigishu Raja*' in his foreign policy for the total destruction of the enemy, the acquisition of all his powers, the expansion and enrichment of the state's resources. In his opinion, an increase in arm strength is not enough for the king. He must immediately show prudence in formulating and implementing shrewd foreign policy.

The '*Mandala* theory' (Circle of Kings) must be discussed in order to be fully informed about foreign policy. As an important royal duty Kautilya emphasized on the occupation of foreign lands and the expansion of the scope of state affairs. In front of '*Vijigishu Raja*', that is the aspirant conqueror being at the centre, Kautilya speaks of five kings who are: Enemy (*Ari*), Conquerer's Ally (*Mitra*), Enemy's Ally (*Ari-Mitra*), Ally's Ally (*Mitra-Mitra*), Enemy's Ally's Ally (*Ari-Mitra-Mitra*), depending on the contiguity of territories.

1. *Ari*: The King of a kingdom situated on either side of the borders of the kingdom of '*Vijigishu Raja*' is called Enemy (Ari), since the King of the frontier kingdom is the natural enemy of 'Vijigishu Raja'.
2. *Mitra*: The King's kingdom, located on the border of the kingdom of enemy (Ari) is the natural enemy of Ari, but the natural ally of '*Vijigishu Raja*'. That is why this King has been called an ally
3. *Ari-mitra*: The adjoining king of the allied king's kingdom is the natural enemy of the allied king. Therefore, this king is the natural ally of the enemy (Ari) and '*Vijigishu*' is the ally of the enemy (*Ari*) of the king.
4. *Mitra-Mitra*: The king whose kingdom is situated on the frontier of the king's enemy's ally (*Ari-Mitra*) is the king's natural friend. So it is the ally's ally (*Mitra-Mitra*) of the '*Vijigishu Raja*'. The King whose kingdom is situated on the border of the kingdom of *Mitra-Mitra* is the natural friend of *Ari-Mitra* (enemy's ally); so he is *Ari-Mitra-Mitra* of the *Vijigishu Raja*. Out of the 5 Kings, mentioned by Kautilya in

front of the *Vijigishu Raja*, 2 Kings are friends of the '*Vijigishu Raja*' and 3 kings are the enemies of '*Vijigishu Raja*'.

As per the scheme of Kautilya if we shift from the frontal configuration to the rear side area, we shall find "*parsnigraha* (the rearward enemy), then *akranda* (rearward friend who can come forward to help the *vijigisu* at call), *parsnigrahasara* (friend and ally of rearward enemy) and *akrandasara* (friend and ally of rearward friend)." Kautilya also speaks of "the *madhyama* king who is close to both the *vijigisu* and his *ari*, able to show his greater strength to either and lastly comes the *udasina* king (most powerful neutral king, very high-placed in strength and resources)" (Basak 1967). But was this conceptual map merely a work of theoretical exercise, perhaps not, because in Kautilya we find equal emphasis on practical knowledge insofar as he had spoken of three kinds of power namely "*mantra- sakti* (the king's power of deliberation with his ministers and priests conversant with the affairs of the state), *prabhusakti* (his power due to adequate possession of treasury and army) and *utsahasakti* (his personal power of giving encouragement and energy) and their corresponding *siddhis* (successes)" (Basak 1967).

Compared to the present scenario no doubt Kautilya's scheme was simplistic. But the penetrating view that transpired from his diplomatic expedients hinged on subtle power calculation that sometimes we tend to naively gloss over. Rather in our dealings with our neighboursw sometimes we have behaved in a benign and altruistic manner notwithstanding the perception by all of India's neighbours that India was hegemonic in South Asia. Such a view of India's neighbours is oblivious of great human tragedies which India had to suffer for partition in 1947. However, it is an irony of the situation that most of the well-admired professionals within the South Bloc are simply "Kautilyan rather than Ashokan in style" but, in practice, our prioritization of values and our rhetoric have always been overtly high- sounding and idealistic, be that Nenhruvian toolkit of *Panchsheel* or Gujral doctrine or of late, Modi's Neighbourhood First policy. That is why, we perceive the necessity of pragmatism and balance to replace hitherto ambivalence in India's foreign policy in the face of very assertive power structure of which broadly all members including India's neighbours are inextricably connected. So, clarity of position is very important and from that perspective, it is foolhardy to think that we seek to conquer new territory and hence trying to draw upon Kautilyan discourse with assiduous interest. Rather, re-reading Kautilya in the context of Chinese imperious design is not to be construed as 'playing fiddle by Nero while Rome was burning', but to stretch out our strategic thought to prevent the enemy from encroaching on our land. Clearly to India if China resembles *Ari* in the frontal configuration then Pakistan's position in India's west and harbouring "the belief that India was bent on undoing Partition and incorporating Pakistan back into Indian fold" makes it similar to *parsnigraha* (i.e. the rearward enemy). So, what we probably get from Kautilya's *Mandala* theory is a kind of premonition that in case of China's offensive or intrusion on Indian territory, there is a likelihood that Pakistan being India's arch enemy, might also attack India from the western sector. Already we are aware that India's western border stretching up to Kashmir is the most militarized sector. Thus, in case of eventuality of Chinese attack in Ladakh or as a light scuffle has already occurred in Sikkim's Naku la, it might open up or tension escalation might provoke Pakistan also to engage with a two-front war with India. The point is how we are prepared because it is not simply the question of accepting the gauntlet as the then army chief now the Chief of our Defense Staff Bipin Rawat once said that "India must be prepared for two-front war along its northern and western fronts". Such a war especially from Pakistan now armed with tactical nuclear weapons (TNW) and mastering the art of employing non- state actors particularly in Kashmir where new insurgent groups have started surfacing like The Resistance Front (i.e. TRF See report published in the Print on 16 April 2020) which are more advanced than its predecessor Lashkar-e-Taiba (LeT) might complicate the situation to the hilt. In the words of Narendra Kumar, senior fellow, CLAWS, New Delhi, "the philosophy of unrestricted war followed by China is omni-directional and has the potential of confrontation in the battlefield as well as in the cyber, information and economic spheres. India has been the target of the irregular and unrestricted warfare capabilities of Pakistan and China. The hybrid threat will be more pronounced in the future as China consolidates its presence..." (CLAWS Journal, Summer 2017).

So, the Indian state has to realize the complexity of 'hybrid war' in a future scenario of 'borderless battlefield' which cannot be fought simply on the basis of military deployment as usually happens in case of conventional warfare. Such wars are highly destabilizing for society and economy because once started it has a tendency to drag on like "no war, no peace situation".

But what a wonder that in Kautilya's writing we find reference of treacherous war or *kuta-yuddha* as well as that of secret war to which we can relate today's diffusion of the concept of warfront and battle. No doubt, Kautilya was very farsighted to conceive of such a war or sabotage which might start by plunging the state into a state of chaos to the advantage of the opportunist enemy to march forward to seize the entire geographical tract or part of it. In that case it might become very difficult to regain the control out of the state of turbulence or initial mistake creating spill-over effect. Of course, we don't know what exactly the design of China is but its gambit in Ladakh at a time when the entire country is worried with infection curve going up is indicative of its malign motive since the disputed land strip happens to be 'a virtually uninhabited high-altitude wasteland', hence an ominous signal no doubt. As per reports 'China's PLA has captured more than 60 square kilometers of Indian patrolled territory in May 2020 and their troops now has blocked access to several Indian patrolling points along the LAC in eastern Ladakh' (https://thekashmirwalla.com/2020/06/china-has-captured-more-than-60-sq-kms-of-indian-patrolled-territory-in-the-last-month/html viewed on 2 June 2020). According to Ashok Sharma of Associated Press, the root of the problem lies in 'China's objection to India's action to building a road through Ladakh's Galwan Valley connecting the region to an airstrip, possibly sparking its move to assert control over territory along the border that is not clearly defined in places (https://thediplomat.com/2020/05/whats-behind-the-latest-india- china-border-tensions/html viewed on 1 June 2020). Yet, some other studies suggest that it is very intriguing to bet how far this Chinese move is 'a bid to expand the territorial claim' or a calculated move to safeguard its deeply-entrenched 'economic interests in the region'. It has been already surmised by Shyam Saran, former foreign secretary of India (Bandyopadhyay and Nag NIICE commentary, May 2020).

The immediate context in which this border row has erupted is also very significant because it is a pointer to growing Chinese unease in the wake of the Covid scenario in which the Anglo-American center of post-Cold War hegemony is out to ostracize Beijing in the international realm. This is vituperative no doubt, but the unilateral Chinese muscle flexing seems very contrived move to divert the attention of the world off from China's liability about the spreading of Corona Virus for which revenge had to be taken. But if we deeply probe we would also discover China's provocation in the recent Kalapani-Lipu-Lekh event in which Nepal upped the ante against India. It was clear from the statement of India's army Chief Manoj Naravane that 'Nepal may have raised the issue at the behest of someone else' (The Hindu, 15 May 2020). It therefore seems no surprised move on the part of Nepal but an underwater plot hatched well in advanced to be used purposely at this moment of vulnerability to put pressure and target India alone when the nation is struggling hard to mitigate a grave health emergency. The suspicion gets apparently confirmed since Nepal remains completely quiet on China even though both China and India have been "referring to Lipu-Lekh Pass as one of their trading points since 1954" (Nayak 2015).

So, it is high time that India should think of her foreign policy strategy vis-à-vis China because 'China's territorial claims and counter- claims have always cast a shadow over Sino-Indian relations and also because their mutual relations are one of the most watched relationship that will shape the Asian century and indeed global geo-politics' (Chakraborty 2014). There is no gainsaying the fact that China's rise and growing assertiveness is infusing lot of stir in India's neighbourhood. So, in this context can we think of applying four elements of Kautilyan diplomacy?

'*Saam, Daam, Danda* and *Bhed*' is by far the most practical idea applied by Vedic kings since time immemorial which remains practical even to this day. *Saam Neeti*: When disagreements arrive, and are not substantially settled, conflicts grow. Identifying and allaying disagreements is the object of *Saam*. It means paying attention to your adversary's argument and understanding his/her perspective. *Daam Neeti*: People work for money, incentives, recognition, awards etc. Chanakya suggests rewarding people sufficiently in order to get the work done. Organizations decide to facilitate by cash or kind, depending upon the policy formulated. *Danda Neeti*: Chanakya says "King with rod becomes a terror. A king with mild rod is despised; king just with rod is honored". Many employees may not show sign of improvement from above methods of motivations in spite of constant follow up. If neither reward nor incentive brings them out of lethargy, punishment is stronger option, but need to be used very intelligently. Punishment is always prescribed for view to improve, not to deteriorate. *Bhed Neeti*: Much abused *neeti* denoting divide and rule, which according to Chanakya is something very important. When no weapon works, then this hard option, though not encouraged at all, is final step.

All of the above mentioned *neeti* goes in a sequence, starting with *Saam Neeti*, if this fails then there is a need to move to *Daam Neeti* and so on. The final step being the *Bhed Neeti* and it is observed in almost all cases that results are attained or seem to be attained if we follow the above principles. The theory has its relevance in contemporary era. The concept of Chanakya *Neeti* must be understood in a broader sense to help in improvement of interests and not deterioration.

Identifying and allaying disagreements is the object of the '*Saam*' or 'patience'. But for Kautilya, patience doesn't mean absolute submission to the whims and fancies of one's adversary. Rather it means paying attention to opponent's capability, argument and understanding their perspective or objective. So here we need a grand diplomacy of sheer intelligence on the part of the nation. 'Gujral Doctrine' is an example of this policy. India advocated a conscious policy of conciliation with neighbors, absolutely without any use of force and settling all pending issues by negotiation, unilateral gestures of goodwill without waiting for reciprocity from smaller states and attempting to move away from fixed position to examine alternatives when an issue seemed intractable. Of late, India is slowly realizing Gujral's desire of expanding his four pronged doctrine for the extended neighborhood that encompasses the Asia pacific region also. Over the past few decades '*Dam*' is getting prominence in Indian foreign policy. India's aid diplomacy towards South Asian neighbors has been driven by economic, historical and political reasons. Development aid to foreign countries not only serves economic objectives but also as a strategic tool. And the neighborhood is the biggest recipient of aid from India in sync with New Delhi's vision of 'neighborhood first' diplomacy. But China too is doing some charitable activities or the act of '*Dana*' in favour of Pakistan. India needs to pay attention to this practical *Dana* logic of the Chinese as India has been cautious that CPEC is nothing but China's debt diplomacy. '*Bheda*' means divide and rule. But the trouble with covert action is that it invites similar retaliation and the probability of backlash which might turn into a spiral prone to escalate rapidly beyond the control of the original handlers. The Americans know this too well after their involvement in Afghanistan boomeranged in the 1990s. But there is a constructive way of looking at this policy. This can open an opportunity for shaping India – Pakistan relations by responding to what the people of Pakistan want and thereby making sense of humanitarian ground to facilitate Indian intervention as it happened way back in 1971. So, '*Danda*' or coercive force is another super-efficient policy that can change geo- politics to tilt the balance in some direction or can act to exact compliance. But such compliance is temporary because stability has never been static. India – China recent standoff is an example of this approach. According to Kautilya, the assessment of the domestic situation derived from internal intelligence should indicate whether a remedial approach or a suppressive approach should be adopted by the state when threats to domestic security are observed. But a grand strategy is vital and indispensable for the external security of the state. Here two prime points are to be noted: first, collecting information about foreign states be they hostile, friendly disposed or neutral is very crucial. Secondly, covert actions against competing or opponent states may be contemplated. Whenever political tensions and instability start, the diplomats should use local agents of influence to exacerbate tensions and to give covert support to treacherous persons and groups as to further weaken and discredit the established governance. And very interestingly, if an armed conflict looms, the nation should use secret agents to weaken the morale to the target leadership and people as well as the combat power of the armed forces through sabotage operations and 'psychological warfare'. In assessing the situation of a competing adversary, or allied state, Kautilya suggests spectrum of available policy options known as '*shadgunya concept*'. According to Kautilya, in a given situation a state must choose between the six more or less foreign policy options-i. *Sandhi* or peace, ii. *Vigraha* or war (similarly Clausewitz proposed war as a continuation of policy), *iii. Asana* or neutrality, iv. *Yana* or war preparation, v. *Samshrya* or alliance building and vi. *Dvaidhibhava* or a diplomatic double game.

Thus, in spite of the vast discrepancy in the level of technology at large and spying technologies in particular in between Indian antiquity and the present, the fundamentals of foreign policy have not substantially changed, just as the nature and survival value of political communities like India have persisted through the ages up to the globalized world of twenty first century. Consequently, the drive for and rationale of diplomatic activities and essence of human wellbeing and intelligence as a phenomenon serving the state have remained essentially unaltered since the time Arthashastra was written. Though India may attempt to fashion for itself a new international identity through its engagement with all major powers, it can't wish away the realities of its difficult continental geography. So, its terrains however difficult should always be guarded well and hence risk-mapping is very important task of national security. So, it requires a distribution along High-risk to Low-risk trajectory where China or Pakistan would always be interested to intervene to wrest the control out of India's hand and if they can do it successfully then the geo-political balance would obviously be tilted in their favour. To India, on the other hand, the best option is to maintain the status quo, but not in a static way. So, it requires India to deploy force and prop up its defence and even to explore 'war-fighting methods'. As India is moving now on twin tracks, that is to 'send signals to Beijing to engage diplomatically to sort out the row while also trying to expand diplomatic efforts towards Australia to ramp up defence cooperation 'to share access to each other's military bases' as a message meant to restrain China. No doubt it shows India is keeping the options open. Yet, this is not sufficient because India might have to depend on its own force as in the past and simultaneously she would be required to do constant nurturing of the camaraderie with smaller neighbours.

Only then in terms of Kautilya's understanding of statecraft based on the interrelationship of intelligence and grand strategy, can it be possible to win over the highly respected '*rakshasa*'. Kautilya, as on a chessboard talks of dynamic and innovative moves with friends and foes in which military option, material capability, non-material elements like command and doctrine, both internal and external are very crucial. We can put forward our wish as expressed by Kautilya that for the sake of security we need to develop and broaden our strategic plan for future although often in reality we tend to think in facile manner that more military power is the key to accumulate more power and prestige. Apparently the present government of India may be following such a muscular policy but according to Ravish Tiwari of *India Today* 'The Modi doctrine' draws upon the ideas of ***Samman*** (i.e. national pride), ***Samvaad*** (i.e. intense diplomatic engagement), to seek ***Samriddhi*** (i.e. greater economic prosperity), ***Suraksha*** (i.e. national, regional and global security through military and diplomatic engagements) and above all, to revive ***Sanskriti*** and ***Sabhyata*** (i.e. cultural and civilizational linkages). Given such a grand projection, the frame of India's overall foreign policy or neighbourhood policy that is unfolding with a mix of maturity and altruism in the context of the Covid-19 pandemic cannot be simply couched as a narrow conflict model but it is rather a veritable neo-hegemonic one with broader Kautilyan dream and resilience.

Bibliography

Books

Basak, Radhagobinda (1967), Some Aspects of Kautilya's Political Thinking, University of Burdwan, Burdwan, India.

Rangarajan, L. N (1992), Koutilya The Arthashastra, Penguin Books, India.

Rich, Bruce.(2008). To upload the world: The message of Ashoka and Kautilya for 21st Century, New Delhi, Viking.

Boesche, Roger,(2003), The First Great Politiical Realist: Kautilya and his Arthashastra, New Yorrk, Lexington Books.

Journals

Kumar, Narendra (2017), War Beyond Rules: Hybrid War and India's Preparedness, CLAWS Journal, Summer 2017.

Bandyopadhyay, Manas Mukul and Nag, Gouri Sankar (May 2020), From Tension Escalation to Thaw: Implications of China's Highhandedness in Ladakh, The NIICE Insight, Vol. I, Issue 5, Kathmandu, Nepal (p 130-132)

Chakraborty, Pinak Ranjan (2014), India's Foreign Policy in the Neighbourhood, Indian Foreign Affairs Journal, Vol.9, No.2, April-June 2014 (p138-153).

Liebig, Michael (2014), Kautilya Arthashastra- A classic text of statecraft and an untapped Political Science resource, South Asian and Comparative Politics, Heidelberg Papers, 74.

Websites consulted

https://thediplomat.com/2020/05/whats-behind-the-latest-india-china-border-tensions/html viewed on 1 June 2020

https://thekashmirwalla.com/2020/06/china-has-captured-more-than-60-sq-kms-of-indian-patrolled-territory-in-the-last-month/html viewed in 2 June 2020

Nayak, Nihar, R (2015), Controversy Over Lipu Lekh Pass: Is Nepal's Stance Politically Motivated? IDSA Comment (Accessed from https://idsa.in/idsacomments/ControversyoverLipu-LekhPass_nnayak_080615 viewed on June 4, 2020)

Newspapers

"New Kailash-Mansarovar road: Nepal may have raised issue at someone else's behest", says Army Chief Viewed from *The Hindu*, 15 May 2020

(https://www.thehindu.com/news/national/new-kailash-mansarovar-road-nepal-may-have-raised-issue-on-someone-elses-behest-says-army-chief/article31590732.ece viewed on 25 May 2020).

3

Pandemics: Challenges and Human Survival

— Squadron Leader Toolika Rani (retd)

Abstract

Infectious diseases have always been a threat to human existence, however urbanization, globalization, rapid transportation and global trade have magnified their fatality quotient multifold. The paper delves into the multifarious challenges pandemics present, the institutional measures developed to tackle these, their efficacy, the controversies surrounding them since ages, the efforts in the face of Covid-19 and the way forward. It utilizes the insights from historical pandemics to perceive the present onslaught and suggests a vision to ensure a multilateral, combined and coherent response and prevention of occurrence of future pandemics.

Key words: Pandemic, historical, urbanization, globalization, Covid-19

"Everybody knows that pestilences have a way of recurring in the world; yet somehow we find it hard to believe in ones that crash down on our heads from a blue sky."

— Author and Philosopher Albert Camus, The Plague, 1948

Despite significant medical progress over the last centuries, infectious diseases still represent significant threats to modern societies. While some have been fought successfully and are only found within a few geographical areas (endemics), others have the ability to spread quickly from an initially limited outbreak, becoming epidemics or pandemics.[1] As per the World Bank Report, pandemics are large-scale outbreaks of infectious disease that can greatly increase morbidity and mortality over a wide geographic area and cause significant economic, social, and political disruption.[2] Key features of a pandemic include wide geographic extension, disease movement, novelty, severity, high attack rates and explosiveness, minimal population immunity, infectiousness and contagiousness.[3] Evidence suggests that the likelihood of pandemics has increased over the past century because of increased global travel and integration, urbanization, changes in land use, and greater exploitation of the natural environment.[4] OECD, among others, sees a severe pandemic as a top global catastrophic risk, one that is higher than terrorism risk. It would bring shared misery, economic decline, and societal disruptions on a global scale, with the poor and those in fragile states hit the hardest.[5]

Significant policy attention has focused on the need to identify and limit emerging outbreaks that might lead to pandemics and to expand and sustain investment to build preparedness and health capacity. Despite these improvements, significant gaps and challenges exist in global pandemic preparedness. Multiple outbreaks, notably the 2014 West Africa Ebola epidemic, have exposed gaps related to the timely detection of disease, availability of basic care, tracing of contacts, quarantine and isolation procedures, and preparedness outside the health sector, including global coordination and response mobilization.[6] The spread of Covid-19 has once again revealed the vulnerability of the human race and highlighted the need to evolve measures to avoid such pandemics in future.

A Timeline of Historical Pandemics

Disease and illnesses have plagued humanity since the earliest days. However, the marked shift to agrarian communities increased the scale and spread of these diseases dramatically. Widespread trade created new opportunities for human and animal interactions that sped up such epidemics. Malaria, tuberculosis, leprosy, influenza, smallpox, and others first appeared during these early years. The more civilized humans became with larger cities, more trade routes, and increased contact with different populations of people, animals, and

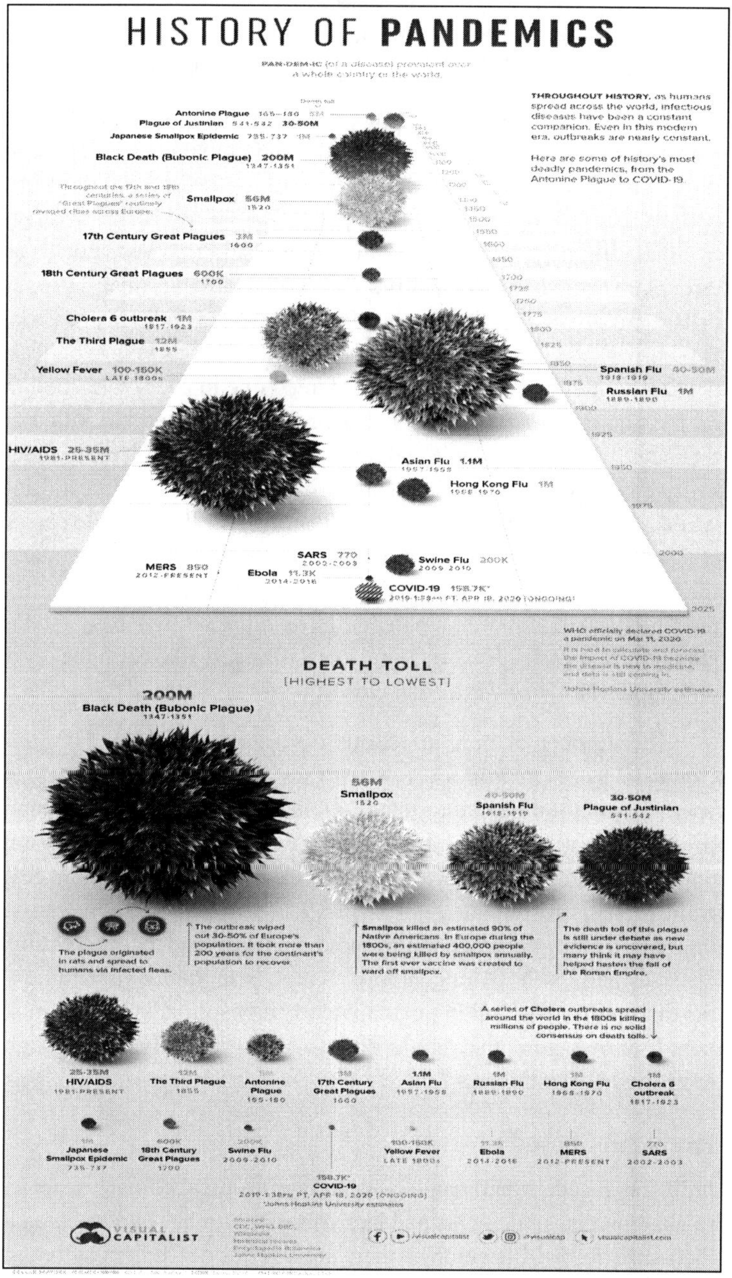
HISTORY OF PANDEMICS
THROUGHOUT HISTORY, as humans spread across the world, infectious diseases have been a constant companion. Even in this modern era, outbreaks are nearly constant.
Here are some of history's most deadly pandemics, from the Antonine Plague to COVID-19.
Antonine Plague 165–180 5M
Plague of Justinian 541–542 30–50M
Japanese Smallpox Epidemic 735–737 1M
Black Death (Bubonic Plague) 200M 1347–1351
Smallpox 56M 1520
17th Century Great Plagues 3M 1600
18th Century Great Plagues 600K 1700
Cholera 6 outbreak 1M 1817–1923
The Third Plague 12M 1855
Yellow Fever 100–150K LATE 1800s
Spanish Flu 40–50M 1918–1919
Russian Flu 1M 1889–1890
HIV/AIDS 25–35M 1981–PRESENT
Asian Flu 1.1M 1957–1958
Hong Kong Flu 1M 1968–1970
SARS 770 2002–2003
MERS 850 2012–PRESENT
Ebola 11.3K 2014–2016
Swine Flu 200K 2009–2010
COVID-19 158.7K* 2019–1:38PM PT, APR 18, 2020 (ONGOING)
DEATH TOLL
[HIGHEST TO LOWEST]
200M Black Death (Bubonic Plague) 1347–1351
56M Smallpox 1520
40–50M Spanish Flu 1918–1919
30–50M Plague of Justinian 541–542
The plague originated in rats and spread to humans via infected fleas.
The outbreak wiped out 30–50% of Europe's population. It took more than 200 years for the continent's population to recover.
Smallpox killed an estimated 90% of Native Americans. In Europe during the 1800s, an estimated 400,000 people were being killed by smallpox annually. The first ever vaccine was created to ward off smallpox.
The death toll of this plague is still under debate as new evidence is uncovered, but many think it may have helped hasten the fall of the Roman Empire.
A series of Cholera outbreaks spread around the world in the 1800s killing millions of people. There is no solid consensus on death tolls.
25–35M HIV/AIDS 1981–PRESENT
12M The Third Plague 1855
5M Antonine Plague 165–180
3M 17th Century Great Plagues 1600
1.1M Asian Flu 1957–1958
1M Russian Flu 1889–1890
1M Hong Kong Flu 1968–1970
1M Cholera 6 outbreak 1817–1923
1M Japanese Smallpox Epidemic 735–737
600K 18th Century Great Plagues 1700
200K Swine Flu 2009–2010
100–150K Yellow Fever LATE 1800s
11.3K Ebola 2014–2016
850 MERS 2012–PRESENT
770 SARS 2002–2003
158.7K* COVID-19 2019–1:38PM PT, APR 18, 2020 (ONGOING)
VISUAL CAPITALIST
/visualcapitalist
@visualcap
visualcapitalist.com

ecosystems, the more likely pandemics would occur. A visual representation of the timeline of major pandemics is given above.[7]

The plague of Justinian struck in the 6th Century and killed as many as 50 million people, perhaps half the global population at the time. The Black Death of the 14th Century caused by the same pathogen killed up to 200 million people. Smallpox killed as many as 300 million people in the 20th Century alone, even though an effective vaccine, the world's first had been available since 1796. 50 to 100 million people died in the 1918 influenza pandemic, numbers that surpass the death toll of World War-I, which was being fought at the same time. The 1918 flu virus infected one in every three people on the planet. HIV pandemic still lacks a vaccine, and has killed an estimated 32 million people and infected 75 million, with more added every day. Malaria has stalked humanity for thousands of years, and while death tolls have dropped significantly over the past 20 years, it still snuffs out nearly half a million people every year. Covid-19 marks the return of a very old and familiar enemy. Throughout history, nothing has killed more human beings than the viruses, bacteria and parasites that cause disease. Not natural disasters like earthquakes or volcanoes. Not war – not even close.[8]

The number of new infectious diseases like SARS, HIV and Covid-19 has increased fourfold over the past century as in past 50 years, population has more than doubled. This means more human beings to get infected and to infect others, especially in densely populated cities. We have more livestock now and viruses can leap from animals to human. As Covid-19 is painfully demonstrating, interconnected global economy both helps spread new infectious diseases and, with its long supply chains, is uniquely vulnerable to the disruption. The ability to get to nearly any spot in the world in 20 hours, allows new diseases to emerge and grow when they might have died out in the past.[9]

Pandemics in India

India has faced several pandemics and her tropical climate, seasonal rains, crowded settlements and lack of sanitation have contributed in their spread. Notable amongst them are a series of Cholera outbreaks from 1817-1899, Bombay Plague epidemic 1896 which created a lot of social and political frenzy, Influenza 1918, Polio (1970-1990) which was successfully erased in 2014, Small Pox (1974) in which India contributed about 85% of cases worldwide, SARS (2003), Chikungunya (2006), Dengue (2006), H1N1 Flu (2009), Swine Flu (2015), and Nipah (2018).[10]

Virus as Mass Killers and War Weapons

Pathogens make effective mass killers because they are self-replicating. This sets them apart from other major threats to humanity. Each bullet that kills in a war must be fired and must find its target. Most natural disasters are constrained by area. But when a virus infects a host, that host becomes a cellular factory to manufacture more viruses. The symptoms created by an infectious pathogen such as sneezing, coughing or bleeding put it in a position to spread to the next host, and the next, a contagiousness captured in the replication number, **"R0" or R Naught** of a pathogen, or how many susceptible people one sick person can infect. (Imperial College London has estimated the novel coronavirus's R0 at 1.5 to 3.5.) And because human beings move around interacting with other human beings they move the microbes with them. Pandemic risk is driven by the combined effects of **spark risk** (where a pandemic is likely to arise) and **spread risk** (how likely it is to diffuse broadly through human populations).[11]

No wonder militaries have long tried to harness disease as a tool of war. Far more soldiers died of disease than died in combat. A pathogen is a perfectly economical weapon, turning its victims into its delivery system.[12]

Aggravating Factors

Superstitions that gods inflict disease upon those who deserve their wrath, lead to disastrous responses. During Justinian's plague, Byzantine historian Procopius despite tracing its origins to China, and via land and sea trade routes to Egypt, blamed Emperor Justinian, declaring him to be a devil, or invoking God's punishment for his evil ways.[13]

Dense concentrations of population, especially in urban centers, can act as foci for disease transmission and accelerate the spread of pathogens. Social inequality and poverty can increase individual susceptibility to infection. Malnutrition weakens an individual's immune system, while lack of clean water and adequate sanitation amplify transmission rates.[14]

Globalization and the growing international movement has increased pandemic risk.[15] Pandemic amnesia and collective myopia in people, governments and organizations are pervasive. People don't think about their family, friends and communities being the source of infection. Each occurrence tends to be treated as a one-off surprise. Bristow (2012) has suggested that since the European and American medical professionals were powerless in the face of the 1918 flu, they omitted it from their professional discourse. History textbooks with twenty pages on World War I have barely one paragraph on the 1918 flu pandemic.

Health sector has inherent bias toward present diseases and pandemics are a very low priority. Developing countries struggle to cope with already existing health problems. Budgets for pandemic preparedness are the first to be cut even in high-income countries. Professional and institutional divides among animal health and human health is another reason for mismanagement of health risks. Necessary communications and collaboration do not occur readily in an emergency, because generally veterinary services are far weaker and less funded than human health departments.[16]

Consequences of Pandemics

Though pandemics originate as a health problem, their consequences don't remain limited just to public health. The impact is wide and long lasting across the entire spectrum of human existence, including the economic, social and psychological areas and their associated fallouts.

Health Impact

When pandemics cause large morbidity and mortality, they are likely to overwhelm health systems. This coupled with other indirect effects may contribute to a 2.3-fold increase in all-cause mortality. The indirect effects include diversion or depletion of resources to provide routine care and decreased access to routine care resulting from an inability to travel, fear, or other factors. Additionally, fear can lead to an upsurge of the "worried well" seeking unnecessary care, further burdening the system. The availability of health care workers also decreases because of illness, deaths, and fear-driven absenteeism.[17]

Economic Impact

Spread of a virus can have important economic implications. Total value of losses (including lost income through reductions in the size of the labour force and productivity, increase in absenteeism and, as the result of individual and social measures that interrupt transmission, but disrupt economic activity, and the intrinsic cost of elevated mortality, incurred by a severe pandemic could reach 0.6 % of global income. A 2019 joint report from the World Health Organization (WHO) and the World Bank estimates the impact of such a pandemic upwards, to 2.2 %-4.8 % of global GDP.[18]

United Nations Department of Economic and Social Affairs (DESA) has estimated that the global economy could shrink by up to 1 per cent in 2020 due to the coronavirus pandemic, a reversal from the previous forecast of 2.5 per cent growth. It said that Covid-19 is disrupting global supply chains and international trade. With nearly 100 countries closing national borders during the past month, the movement of people and tourism flows have come to a halt. As businesses lose revenue, unemployment is likely to increase sharply, transforming a supply-side shock to a wider demand-side shock. It warns that the adverse effects of prolonged economic restrictions in developed economies will soon spill over to developing countries via trade and investment channels. A sharp decline in consumer spending in the European Union and the United States will reduce imports of consumer goods from developing countries. Meanwhile, the decline in commodity-related revenues and a reversal of capital flows are increasing the likelihood of debt distress for many nations.[19] All sectors of the economy face disruption, potentially leading to shortages, rapid price increases for staple goods, and economic stresses for households, private firms, and governments.[20]

Social Impact

Restriction on movement, closure of public places, and instructions from government, doctors and media for social distancing impacts social behavior. This may result in psychological changes such as aversion from office, fear, unwillingness to travel, and meet people, reduction in social trust affecting economy. Increase in domestic violence, depression, anxiety, suicidal tendencies may arise.

Preparedness against Pandemics

"Preparedness, including for potential pandemics, requires coordination and management of complex relationships across different sectors and between international, national, and local actors. We must work together in support of all societies, in ways that reflect the interests of all people for whom preparations are being made. A community-based One Health approach is essential for reducing the risks to people that emerge at the interfaces between animals, humans, and ecosystems."

—UN System Influenza Coordinator David Nabarro, 2013[21]

Preparedness measure include the following:

- Public health infrastructure capable of identifying, tracing, managing, and treating cases
- Adequate physical and communications infrastructure to channel information and resources
- Fundamental bureaucratic and public management capacities
- Capacity to mobilize financial resources to pay for disease response and weather the economic shock of the outbreak
- Ability to undertake effective risk communications.[22]

Countries may use the World Health Organization's Joint External Evaluation mechanism to identify their current state and possible needs. It evaluates each country's preparedness in four main areas, i.e. **prevention** (which includes national legislation, policy and financing; international health regulation coordination, communication and advocacy, antimicrobial resistance, zoonotic diseases food safety, biosafety and biosecurity and immunisation); **detection** (through national laboratory systems, real-time surveillance, reporting and workforce development); **response** (including emergency response operations, linking public health and security authorities, medical countermeasures and personnel deployment as well as risk communication); and **other** related hazards and points of entry.[23]

Quarantine: A Historical Way to Check Transmission

The term Quarantine originated from Italian word Quaranta giorni meaning 40 days and the practice has been in existence since 14th century. During the plague epidemic of 1347–1352 in Italy a sanitary cordon was imposed by armed guards along transit routes and access points to cities. Separation between healthy and infected persons was accomplished through camps. Quarantine was first introduced in 1377 in Dubrovnik on Croatia's Dalmatian Coast, and the first permanent plague hospital (lazaretto) was opened by Venice in 1423.[24] In 1830-32 when Cholera the "Asiatic disease" reached Europe and the United States, travelers returning from a place where cholera was present were quarantined.

In 1911, Encyclopedia Britannica emphasized that "the old sanitary preventive system of detention of ships and men" was "a thing of the past". However, nations were forced to implement it again in response to the 1918 influenza pandemic. Army Medical officers isolated soldiers with symptoms. Disease-containment strategies, including the closure of schools, churches, theaters and suspension of public gatherings were implemented. In Paris, a sporting event, in which 10,000 youths were to participate, was postponed. Physicians encouraged measures like respiratory hygiene and social distancing.[25]

Traditional intervention measures were resurrected in response to SARS, which originated in China, in 2003, and spread along air-travel routes. In Canada, public health authorities asked persons who might have been exposed to SARS to voluntarily quarantine themselves. In China, police cordoned off buildings, organized checkpoints, and even installed cameras in private homes.

More than half a millennium since quarantine became the core of a multicomponent strategy for controlling pandemics, it has been an essential way to reduce contact between the sick and the susceptible. In the absence of pharmaceutical interventions, such measures help contain infection, delay the spread, avert terror and death, and maintain the infrastructure of society. However, these strategies have always been much debated, perceived as intrusive, and accompanied in every age and under all political regimes by an undercurrent of suspicion, distrust, and riots. They continue to raise a variety of political, economic, social, and ethical issues. The historical perspective helps in understanding the extent to which panic, social stigma and prejudice, can frustrate public health efforts to control the spread. But due to the globalized media, fear, alarm, and panic can spread farther and faster. Therefore, it is required to employ vigilant attention to avoid causing prejudice and intolerance. Public trust must be gained through regular, transparent, and comprehensive communications that balance the risks and benefits of public health interventions.[26]

India's efforts against Covid-19

At the news of Covid-19 spread in Wuhan, India reacted with considerable alacrity, evacuated its citizens, and kept them in 14 days' quarantine. Thermal checking of the passengers returning from Covid incidence countries was carried out and the symptomatic people quarantined. After a one day 'Janata Curfew' on 20 March 2020, India announced a 21 day's lockdown from 22 March which was extended further till 03 May to prevent the community transmission. To alleviate the hardships of the marginalized sections, Garib Kalyan Yojna with 1.7 Lakh crore was implemented with cash transfers, home delivery of ration and free gas cylinders. Reserve Bank of India infused liquidity in the market to prevent collapse of economy. Prime Minister Narendra Modi kept a continuous communication with people, garnering public co-operation and keeping the morale high in the fight against the pandemic. Technology was widely used to disseminate information regarding preventive measures including Arogya Setu App. Zone mapping of the country with hotspots has been done to seal off these areas while the safe zones may be opened gradually with precautions and continued surveillance. Doctors, health workers, sanitation workers and volunteers have been at the forefront of the response against Covid-19. At international level, India took the lead to organize a virtual SAARC meeting and called for creation of Covid Relief Fund.

Conclusion

Pandemics cause devastation to human lives and livelihoods much as do wars and financial crises. Pandemic prevention and response, therefore, should be treated as an essential tenet of both national and global security, not just as a matter of health.[27] In this context, an International Monetary Fund paper emphasises the importance of (i) investing in improved sanitation, provision of clean water and improved urban infrastructure; (ii) building strong health systems and supporting proper nutrition; (iii) investing in reliable disease surveillance; (iv) collaborating between countries to improve monitoring of Economic impact of epidemics and pandemics outbreaks and increase response readiness.[28]

As organizations and governments around the world ask for citizens to practice social distancing to help reduce the rate of infection, the digital world is allowing people to maintain connections and commerce.[29] In this regard, Prime Minister Modi's emphasis on **AEIOU Model** of commerce, signifying Adaptability, Efficiency, Inclusivity, Opportunity and Universalism is a way forward in the changed circumstances to utilize the available digital opportunities for sustainable development of one and all.

UN Chief Economist Elliot Harris said that the collective goal must be a resilient recovery which puts the planet back on a sustainable track. The UN Department of Economic and Social Affairs advised, "A well-designed fiscal stimulus package, prioritising health spending to contain the spread of the virus and providing income support to households most affected by the pandemic would help to minimise the likelihood of a deep economic recession". It has further asked for a "large-scale, coordinated, comprehensive multilateral response" amounting to at least 10 per cent of global gross domestic product (GDP)."[30]

Advance research in the field of pandemic prevention is the need of the hour for preparedness against the future crisis. The concept of 'Herd Immunity' which propounds that if a larger section of population is immune to the disease it may provide protection to the not vaccinated also, may be explored further. Attention should be paid to mitigate the psychological impacts of the pandemic and control measures.

In this direction the step by Indian Department of Science and Technology to launch SATYAM App to invite proposals to study appropriate intervention of Yoga and meditation in fighting Covid-19 and similar kinds of viruses is praiseworthy. Pandemics show that the human race is interdependent; it swims or sinks together, and therefore, the global efforts shall be to strengthen the weakest link in order to be strong enough to survive and prevent a pandemic.

References

1. Angelos Delivorias and Nicole Scholz, EPRS | European Parliamentary Research Service, Members' Research Service, PE 646.195 – February 2020, p. 1.
2. Dean T. Jamison, Hellen Gelband, Susan Horton, Prabhat Jha, Ramanan Laxminarayan, Charles N., Mock Rachel Nugent, Disease Control Priorities: Improving Health and Reducing Poverty, World Bank Group, Third Edition, Vol. 9, p. 315.
3. Qiu W., Rutherford S., Mao A., Chu C., The Pandemic and its Impacts, Health, Culture and Society Vol. 9–10 (2016–2017) | ISSN 2161-6590 (online) | DOI 10.5195/hcs.2017.221 | http://hcs.pitt.edu, p.3.
4. Dean T. Jamison, Hellen Gelband, Susan Horton, Prabhat Jha, Ramanan Laxminarayan, Charles N., Mock Rachel Nugent, Disease Control Priorities: Improving Health and Reducing Poverty, World Bank Group, Third Edition, Vol. 9, p. 315.
5. Olga Jonas, Pandemic Risk, October 2013, background paper to the World Development Report 2014 on Risk and Opportunity: Managing Risks for Development, p. ii.
6. Dean T. Jamison, Hellen Gelband, Susan Horton, Prabhat Jha, Ramanan Laxminarayan, Charles N., Mock Rachel Nugent, Disease Control Priorities: Improving Health and Reducing Poverty, World Bank Group, Third Edition, Vol. 9, p. 315.
7. Le Pan Nicholas, Visualizing the History of Pandemics, https://www.visualcapitalist.com/history-of-pandemics-deadliest/, March 14, 2020.
8. Walsh Bryan, Covid-19: The history of pandemics, BBC Future, 26 March 2020.
9. Walsh Bryan, Covid-19: The history of pandemics, BBC Future, 26 March 2020.

10. Swetha G., Anantha Eashwar V M., Gopalakrishnan S, Epidemics and Pandemics in India throughout History: A Review Article, Indian Journal of Public Health Research and Development, January 2019, https://www.researchgate.net/publication/336061202_Epidemics_and_Pandemics_in_India_throughout_History_A_Review_Article/link/5dd789b492851c1feda589c2/download
11. Dean T. Jamison, Hellen Gelband, Susan Horton, Prabhat Jha, Ramanan Laxminarayan, Charles N., Mock Rachel Nugent, Disease Control Priorities: Improving Health and Reducing Poverty, World Bank Group, Third Edition, Vol. 9, p. 317.
12. Walsh Bryan, Covid-19: The history of pandemics, BBC Future, 26 March 2020.
13. Le Pan Nicholas, Visualizing the History of Pandemics, https://www.visualcapitalist.com/history-of-pandemics-deadliest/, March 14, 2020.
14. Dean T. Jamison, Hellen Gelband, Susan Horton, Prabhat Jha, Ramanan Laxminarayan, Charles N., Mock Rachel Nugent, Disease Control Priorities: Improving Health and Reducing Poverty, World Bank Group, Third Edition, Vol. 9, p. 317.
15. Olga Jonas, Pandemic Risk, October 2013, background paper to the World Development Report 2014 on Risk and Opportunity: Managing Risks for Development, p. 11.
16. Olga Jonas, Pandemic Risk, October 2013, background paper to the World Development Report 2014 on Risk and Opportunity: Managing Risks for Development, pp. 23-25.
17. Dean T. Jamison, Hellen Gelband, Susan Horton, Prabhat Jha, Ramanan Laxminarayan, Charles N., Mock Rachel Nugent, Disease Control Priorities: Improving Health and Reducing Poverty, World Bank Group, Third Edition, Vol. 9, p. 323.
18. Angelos Delivorias and Nicole Scholz, Economic impact of epidemics and pandemics, Members' Research Service, EPRS | European Parliamentary Research Service, PE 646.195 – February 2020, p. 2.
19. The Economic Times, 02 April 2020, available from:
https://economictimes.indiatimes.com/news/international/business/global-economy-could-shrink-by-almost-1-in-2020-due-to-covid-19-pandemic-united-nations/articleshow/74943235.cms
20. Olga Jonas, Pandemic Risk, October 2013, background paper to the World Development Report 2014 on Risk and Opportunity: Managing Risks for Development, pp. 23-25.
21. Olga Jonas, Pandemic Risk, October 2013, background paper to the World Development Report 2014 on Risk and Opportunity: Managing Risks for Development.
22. Dean T. Jamison, Hellen Gelband, Susan Horton, Prabhat Jha, Ramanan Laxminarayan, Charles N., Mock Rachel Nugent, Disease Control Priorities:

Improving Health and Reducing Poverty, World Bank Group, Third Edition, Vol. 9, p. 320.

23. Angelos Delivorias and Nicole Scholz, Economic impact of epidemics and pandemics, Members' Research Service, EPRS | European Parliamentary Research Service, PE 646.195 – February 2020, p. 6.
24. Eugenia Tognotti, 'Lessons from the History of Quarantine, from Plague to Influenza A', Emerging Infectious Diseases • www.cdc.gov/eid • Vol. 19, No. 2, February 2013, p. 254-255.
25. Eugenia Tognotti, 'Lessons from the History of Quarantine, from Plague to Influenza A', Emerging Infectious Diseases • www.cdc.gov/eid • Vol. 19, No. 2, February 2013, p. 257.
26. Eugenia Tognotti, 'Lessons from the History of Quarantine, from Plague to Influenza A', Emerging Infectious Diseases • www.cdc.gov/eid • Vol. 19, No. 2, February 2013, p. 258-259.
27. Qiu W, Rutherford S, Mao A., Chu C., The Pandemic and its Impacts, Health, Culture and Society Vol 9–10 (2016–2017) | ISSN 2161-6590 (online) | DOI 10.5195/hcs.2017.221 | http://hcs.pitt.edu, p. 8.
28. Angelos Delivorias and Nicole Scholz, Economic impact of epidemics and pandemics, Members' Research Service, EPRS | European Parliamentary Research Service, PE 646.195 – February 2020, p. 6-7.
29. Le Pan Nicholas, Visualizing the History of Pandemics, https://www.visualcapitalist.com/history-of-pandemics-deadliest/, March 14, 2020.
30. The Economic Times, 02 April 2020, available from: https://economictimes.indiatimes.com/news/international/business/global-economy-could-shrink-by-almost-1-in-2020-due-to-covid-19-pandemic-united-nations/articleshow/74943235.cms

4

Ensuring Learner Engagement During Covid-19 Pandemic: Pedagogical Methods for Online Education

— *Dr. Shreya Pathak*

Technology has completely revolutionised the way we think, plan and implement any work. Use of technology has entered every domain of our life and education is not untouched. The outbreak of COVID-19 pandemic and global implementation of complete lockdown to contain its spread has left use of technology as the only viable alternative for the teaching fraternity to mitigate the effect of lockdown on teaching learning process, though Government has been incessantly working on various e-learning platforms and integration of technology in education since few years and MHRD has taken number of ICT initiatives like offering MOOCs through SWAYAM, broadcasting of educational programme through 32 D2H channels of Swayamprabha and Vyas channel of Consortium for Educational Communication prepared in its Media Centres, repository of e-resources and e-books like National Digital Library of India, Shodhganga, Inflibnet, N-List, epgpathshala, egyankosh etc.[1] Its policy is to emphasize on use of technology enabled teaching-learning. Chapter 19 of the Draft National Education Policy 2019 (DNEP) is exclusively dedicated to Technology in Education. The document clearly mentions the objective of use of technology in education,

"*Appropriate integration of technology into all levels of education - to support teacher preparation and development; improve teaching, learning and evaluation processes; enhance educational access to disadvantaged groups; and streamline educational planning, administration and management.*" It talks about establishment of National Education Technology Forum (NETF) with the purpose to leverage best available updated technology and various tools to improve educational outcomes and provide a platform to improve learning, assessment, planning and administration in the field of education.[2]

In the learning space of the students, earlier it was either only physical space that includes classroom set up, laboratories or it was mixture of physical space integrated with digital space, but the present threat of COVID-19 pandemic has created a sudden and complete shift from physical to digital learning spaces with infusion of technology dominantly. Teachers or educators are adopting various teaching learning platforms and tools for imparting education and making every endeavour to smoothly run the teaching-learning process despite many limitations and restrictions. Though digital divide is the major concern of all stakeholders as education is not in blended or flipped classroom mode, but being imparted hundred percent through technology as the medium of communication. Due to this many underprivileged students and others in remote areas with no facility of good network or weak bandwidth are left out from the teaching- learning process. Another issue that educators need to ponder over is that even those students who are equipped with all necessary hardware, skill and network are not being involved in learning process to the level to which teachers are expecting. In the physical classroom setting, teachers could observe those students who were physically present in the class, but mentally not completely engaged. In virtual setting, it is found that most of the students mute their mic and put off their cameras and display their fake presence on the virtual platform. This is coming up as a major concern for EPS community.

The major challenge that is being faced by the educators is to ensure learner engagement during virtual teaching by adopting various pedagogical methods as per the need of the pressing situation. This chapter particularly focuses on and explores various pedagogical methods that can be adopted by teachers to ensure learner engagement not only during virtual classes, but also after classes by assigning various task to ensure active learning, development of various learning domains- cognitive, affective and psychomotor as this will enhance learning skills and enable the teacher to get a feedback of how and to what level the learner has been receptive. Virtual teaching or online teaching can be categorically divided into two types:

1. **Synchronous learning:** An online education that happens in real time. In this type of learning, virtual classes are conducted live through various platforms like live streaming on facebook, youtube, teleconferencing, video-conferencing through applications like zoom cloud meeting, Microsoft teams, Go to meeting, Google meet, cisco webex etc. This mode of teaching-learning allows interactions among all participants on specific time. Face-to-face discussions, clearance of doubts and queries after lecture, immediate feedback of learners, regular interactions with professors, attendance, feel of presence of teacher etc. are the benefits of model of synchronous learning. Learners can view presentations, converse in groups, connect to various e-learning websites. With this it has its own disadvantages. Fixation of time schedule is one of the major issue. This rigidity aggravates the technical issues and difficulties of the learners like availability of network and good bandwidth in a particular time slot, sudden technical problems with hardware and other important equipment and software that is to be used to complete and submit a particular assignment. It also ignores personal problems of the learners like family and health issues where learner is not in a position to attend the class.

2. **Asynchronous learning:** An online mode of teaching where knowledge is imparted by the teacher through various available e-platforms without any interaction on real-time basis. This includes Learning Management System (LMS) like Moodle, Google Classroom, Blackboard Inc, schoology etc. The best

feature of this mode of learning is that it provides complete flexibility to the learners regarding time schedule and learning pace. Learner can attend all the created and existed e-contents like video-lectures and reading materials according to their own time. Since there is no rigidity of time in this learning model, so even if a learner is having weak bandwidth and staying in remote areas, s/he can manage by downloading posted e-contents when bandwidth is good and can use that material later. This model addresses different learning pace of the students. They can watch lecture-videos many times according to their learning pace. These LMS provides platform to conduct quizzes, test and variety of assignment as per need of the course. This learning model, though sounds too good, has its own disadvantages. In the absence of personal touch of the teacher and direct interaction, students may feel isolated. It also does not provide immediate feedback of the learners that teachers generally do get in physical classroom set up simply by seeing the students' expressions and lines on their forehead that reflects their uneasiness and difficulty in understanding the illustrations that teacher is using to elaborately explain various topics. It also fails to provide peer learning and collaborative learning environment. Moreover, these learning platforms fail to address advance learners who do not get that level of motivation and opportunity to show their intellectual qualities through debates, discussions, group activities, follow up questions and discussions after each lecture.

Both the learning models have their own advantages and disadvantages. Its blended use can address the needs of the learners and would also enable the teacher to establish direct connection and interaction with the students that gives them a sense of belonging. Other than this, few pedagogical methods to ensure learner engagement can be adopted in both the online learning models to address the needs of the students depending on the nature of the discipline and topic to be taught. This requires few learner centered strategies to promote active learning and enhance learning experience through use of various available technological tools.

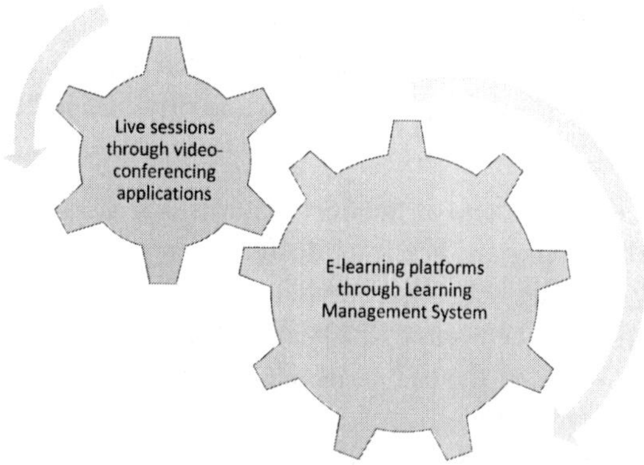

Two Models of Online Learning: Synchronous and Asynchronous

Pedagogical Methods for Synchronous Online Education

While commencing teaching-learning through synchronous model, a teacher should ensure that all the students are aware of the use of e-platform that is being used for classes and various video-conferencing applications like Google meet, Microsoft teams, zoom cloud meetings, go to meeting, cisco webex, skype etc. One should inform about steps to download the applications and necessary features of the application that is being used for classes. Before commencing teaching, it is always preferred to establish a connection between the teacher and the students. A brief introduction of all students is necessary for establishment of smooth learning environment. While teaching a topic, it is always better to prefer use of power point presentation through screen sharing option as this will not only engage the students, but will enable them to jot down the important points that they missed due to weak bandwidth or voice disturbance. Visual memory always do have better retention and easy retrieval from memory compared to auditory memory since the learners mind could easily relate to pictures, graphs, diagrams, objects, images used in presentation by the teacher. This method provides learners of different learning pace to comprehend difficult topics in a simple manner, which in turn improves learner engagement. While teaching, teacher's video should always be on active mode to establish connect with learners. Various animations can be created in presentations using tools like zetings, prezi presentation etc. for lively power points. Use of graphs, charts, mind- mapping, Venn diagram, data in tabular form is an effective pedagogy for conceptual understanding and provides better platform to teach using illustrations.

Live captions is one of the best features that is available in few video-conferencing applications designed especially for teaching purpose. It not only helps those students who have weak bandwidth, but also addresses the needs of the hearing challenged learners. Online white board is one of the best tools to explain concepts and facilitate collaborative work. Video-conferencing applications do have inbuilt whiteboard that can be used through screen sharing option. Other than this there are collaborative online whiteboard applications available with extra features as per the need of the teaching-learning process that work on real time basis like whiteboard.fi, awwapp, web white board etc. While the topic is being taught, students should be encouraged to post their queries in chat box that can be addressed by the end of the session. For this feature of 'chat box' and 'raise hand' should be used. This will establish direct interaction with the learners and will also provide immediate feedback of the classes as the queries reflect the level to which learner has understood the topic.

Blended learning or flipped classroom: In physical set up, one can use various pedagogical methods like problem solving methods, experiential learning, participative learning, which is not easy in online set up. One can explore various technological tools to facilitate and promote collaborative, participative learning, peer-to-peer learning. Assignments and task could be regularly assigned to broaden the learning experience. Students can be divided into groups for group activities that can be done online using tools like Google documents, Padlet, Answer garden etc. Padlet is a free electronic bulletin board for collaborative learning, project work and brainstorming. A teacher can use this tool to create the board, share its link with all the students through chatbox that allows all learners to write and share their ideas, opinion, which can be seen by all. A focus question can also be posted by the teacher on Padlet, share links and videos. It can be used in various innovative ways like creating a board with newspaper clippings on a particular topic. It is a free tool that allows creating atleast three e-boards and also can be downloaded. This not only engages students, but will also enable teachers to get immediate feedback. Answer Garden is another important online tool for brainstorming and collaborative work. One of the best tools for collaborative project work is Google Document that allows many people to work on a single created document at same time from different places. This works on real time basis and can be commented and edited by all those who have been given the right to edit through link sharing by the creator of the document. This online tool also displays the history of all editions, deletions, additions, comments with date and time. It is one of the best available online tools for collaborative project work. It also has many other features available in G suite Marketplace that can be added to document through Add ons option.

Another way to ensure engagement is to use Google earth in live sessions. One can use this tool to show different heritage sites, places, maps, geographical locations, places of strategic importance and other things. It allows 3D vision that gives a glimpse of experiential learning to slight extent and not only makes teaching interesting, but also allows better reception and memory of the learners. Google forms can also be used in various ways in teaching like conducting online surveys for project, focus question, to take attendance of the students, to collect data of the learners so that teacher can have a better understanding and record of all the students, to conduct quizzes, to take feedback of the classes etc. These various tools can be used to identify slow and advanced learners and understand students' profile, which is a challenge for teachers in case of purely online teaching mode during pandemic lockdown.

Use of all these tools allow student centric and activity based teaching that broaden and enhance the learning experience. Learner centric approach focuses mainly on learner and the learning process, rather than the teacher. In this, teachers' role is more of a facilitator. Here the focus of instruction is shifted from teacher to student opposite to that of conventional lecture method.[3] Live sessions can be recorded and shared with the students so that they could refer these videos whenever required. This will allow managing the limitations of synchronous classes to some extent by addressing the needs of the learners who due to one reason or other could not attend the class or are slow learners.

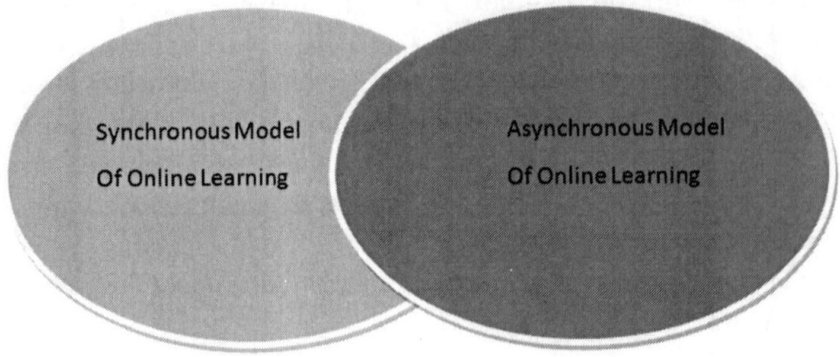

Diagram showing online model of Blended Learning

Pedagogical Methods for Asynchronous Online Education

According to Sofia and Alves from University of Lisbon, "Blended learning meets multiple and differentiated instructional online activities, therefore it has the potential, human and technological, of accommodating students with distinct learning needs."[4] Asynchronous online education mainly uses various online platforms that are provided through Learning Management System (LMS). LMS provides an e-platform that can be used for delivery of a course or programme in an organized way. According to Black et al, LMS enables structured course e-content, organize classes and manage various teaching- learning activities like that of blended learning. It has many technological tools integrated into its system for collaborative, sharing and interactive learning environment.[5] Here learners can see lecture videos, other existing videos, files, e-text, content material, extra reading material, links, assessment, assignment, quizzes etc. There are many popular LMS available like Google Classroom, Moodle, Edmodo, Blackboard Inc., Schoology etc. Google Classroom integrates all google tools within this LMS like Google meet, document, sheet, slides, drive, form, calendar. MS Office 365 A3/A5 package is specially designed keeping in mind educational needs of Higher Education Institutions and integrates all tools of MS Office. Top LMS software are:

(a) Adobe Captivate Prime
(b) Docebo
(c) SAP Litmos LMS
(d) Learn Upon LMS
(e) Asentia LMS

E-contents: These are broadly two types, created and existed that include both videos and text in pdf format. For proper delivery of course/ programme, it is important to focus on the type of video that is being created as per the need of the topic being taught and the nature of the discipline. The teacher must also be aware of use of various tools that are required to create lecture videos. There are types of videos like table-top (used for mathematics, equation or problem solving topics), talking head, slide video, picture in picture (PIP), overhead videos (generally used for displaying practicals). Existing videos can also be shared that are available on SWAYAM through

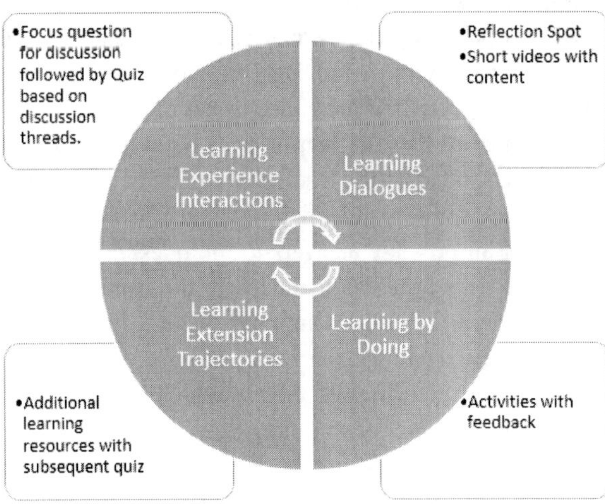

Diagram showing four components of Learner Centric model developed by IIT, Bombay

various courses offered, videos broadcasted through 32 D2H channels of Swayamprabha, Consortium for Educational Communication, Vyas channel etc. For e-text, content can be created or existing content can be shared like those available on various e-learning platforms such as epgpathshala, inflibnet, NLIST, National Digital Library, jstor articles, egyankosh, National Repository of Open Educational Resources (OER). In case of asynchronous classes, learner centric model mainly includes four components that are connected to each other and should be focused while planning the delivery of the course in case of asynchronous education model.[6]

1. **Learning Dialogues (LeDs)**: These are lecture videos of any type- talking head, PIP or slide that includes Reflection spot. It is a point of logical pause where learner is required to answer a question that may enable the learner to reflect on the preceding content, express their thinking, apply concept that they have already learned immediately, do micro- practice. This also provides feedback to the learner. The main purpose of LeD is generally to provide conceptual understanding. This reflection spot is generally in form of one word answer, MCQ or MSQ format. It enhances learner engagement and active learning. Generally these LeDs are of short time duration as in case of long LeDs there are high chances of passive listening. The placement of these reflection spots is at a logical pause point that is decided by the teacher. It can be in the beginning of the lecture or towards the end of the lecture, but it must be followed by all possible answers to the questions with right explanation. This provides feedback to the learners on their own responses and broadens their perspective. It establishes a type of interaction with the learners. The purpose of reflection spot is to end learner disengagement, which is normally seen in monologue content transmission. Since LeDs are preferred to be short videos as these are more engaging and effective. It is always better for a teacher to chunk their main topics into small topics with natural pause points in a lecture and create a series of LeDs on a single topic.
2. **Learning by Doing (LbDs)**: It is a formative assessment activity to check the level of concept attainment by the

learners. This provides immediate application of the knowledge gained and feedback from the learners. This can be in MSQ, MCQ, one word or long answers. For this Google form can be used to create ungraded quizzes. Link of the form can be shared with the learners. These questions must show the right answers after the form is submitted and should also provide feedback as to why a particular answer is correct or reason why answers are wrong so the learner may get a better understanding and can avail the real purpose with which LbD is designed.

3. **Learning Extension Trajectories (LxT)**: These are basically additional learning sources or material that is shared with the learners to have broaden learning experience. This component perfectly addresses the demand of advanced learners, who can explore the source material as per their interest. This can be in form of articles, research papers, videos, websites, reports, surveys, interview etc. These LxTs are followed by few questions in quiz form just to ensure that the learner has gone through the shared material. It should include only those questions answer of which is mentioned in the shared learning material. Generally these questions enable checking and ensure the conceptual understanding of the main topic by the learner. This pedagogy enables the teacher to address the diversity of learners.

4. **Learning Experience Interaction (LxIs)**: In order to promote discussion, enhance peer active and participative learning it is important to establish interaction with all peers. For active participation of all in the discussion and to keep the discussion channelized, one topic or question can be given. This is known as focus question. This question can be of analytical and critical level to motivate active discussion among learners. All this ensures learner engagement, active participation, enables the teacher to identify passive learners and push them, motivate advance learners who can show their intellectual qualities through discussions otherwise there is much fear of isolation in asynchronous model of online education. To address and push the passive listeners, these

discussions can be followed by reflection quiz that is based on these discussions. These discussion threads enable the learners to put and know various perspectives, opinions on a single issue through learner-learner interaction and learner-instructor interaction. All this cultivate peer learning by answering queries of others.

Use of any one online learning model would never fulfill the purpose of education and will also make the teaching-learning process cumbersome as both the models have their own disadvantages. To make an optimum utilization of all the available online resources for education purpose, the best way is to blend both the models and plan teaching and formative assessments according to Bloom's taxonomy where lower level cognitive skills can be developed among students through asynchronous model of online education and higher order thought can be encouraged using synchronous online model of learning by conducting number of activities designed accordingly. While activities are planned in both the learning models, the teacher should avoid cognitive overload.

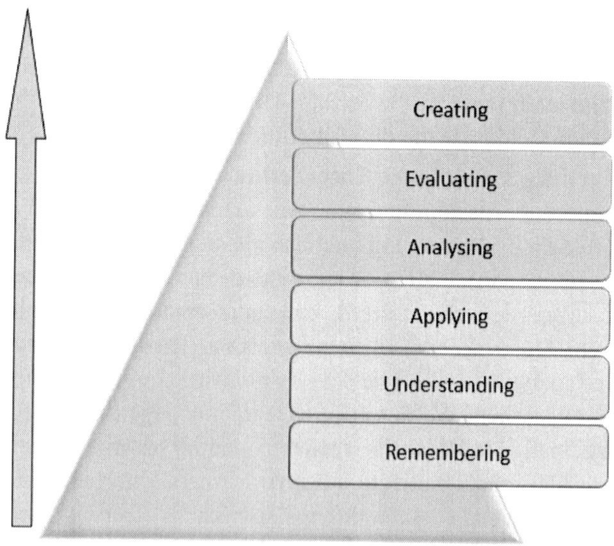

Bloom's Taxonomy Model of Learning showing higher and lower cognitive levels

ICT has turned from optional to essential tool in the changing scenario of lockdown, emerging as the only solution of imparting education and continuing incessant teaching-learning process with smooth interaction between the teachers and the students. The recent pandemic has completely changed the way education is being imparted globally. Technology enhanced learning with teaching-learning methodologies would ensure engagement of learners and provide better learning outcomes through augmentation of active learning. Indubitably, technology has provided us opportunities for active learning, smooth distant communication and collaboration. Though all this has come with major concerns related to EPS community that could not be ignored and has to be dealt with all in tandem effectively. Online education can never replace classroom teaching, but can facilitate it during this pressing time.

References

1. ICT Initiatives of MHRD (e-brochure), Department of Higher Education, MHRD, Government of India, https://mhrd.gov.in/ict-initiatives.
2. Draft National Education Policy 2019, MHRD, Government of India, pp. 339-343. Retrieved on 28.5.2020 https://mhrd.gov.in/sites/upload_files/mhrd/files/Draft_NEP_2019_EN_Revised.pdf
3. Groen, J., & Li, Q. (2005). Achieving the Benefits of Blended Learning within a Fully Online Learning Environment: A Focus on Synchronous Communication. *Educational Technology, 45*(6), 31-37. Retrieved June 11, 2020, from www.jstor.org/stable/44429250
4. Sofia Balula Dias, & José Alves Diniz. (2014). Towards an Enhanced Learning Management System for Blended Learning in Higher Education Incorporating Distinct Learners' Profiles. *Journal of Educational Technology & Society, 17*(1), 307-319. Retrieved June 11, 2020, www.jstor.org/stable/jeductechsoci.17.1.307
5. Black, E. R., Beck, D., Dawson, K., Jinks, S., & DiPietro, M. (2007). The other side of the LMS: Considering implementation and use in the adoption of an LMS in online and blended learning environments. TechTrends, 51(2), pp. 35-39.
6. These components are based on the MOOC course Designing Learner-Centric MOOCs offered on SWAYAM platform under the aegis of NPTEL by Prof. Sridhar Iyer et al, IIT Bombay.

5

Women Self Help Groups: A Powerful Tool to Rebuild Life During and Post Covid-19

— *Prof. Madhu Rajput*

Every situation comes with two facets to it, one is of challenge and the other of opportunity. Adversity, despite bringing in its wake a horde of negative impacts, also encapsulates an opportunity to innovate, to make collective efforts to overcome it and to harness and utilize the latent powers in an individual, community or nation. COVID-19 has presented an unprecedented challenge in front of humanity with all the established notions of existence- be it individual, social, economic, political or cultural norms. With life coming to a complete standstill for a few months and the global linkages snapped suddenly, every entity has been forced to look inwards. The painstakingly created norms of international interactions in various fields had to be discarded and a new way of life had to be envisioned, which rests on the plank of self-dependence. As the crisis got deepened, unusual heroes have come to fore. Faced with a survival challenge, the remarkable ability of human beings to improvise, adapt and innovate has come to the forefront once again. In this context one such unit of our socio- economic fabric which erstwhile existed more as a supplementary entity has garnered praise for its quick adaptation and for its multifarious role in sustaining life amidst such a herculean crisis. These are the almost non-descript Self Help Groups which have suddenly caught attention for their tremendous contribution in not only keeping afloat many a families economically in such hard times, but also emerging as a supplier of essential medical items such as masks, protective clothing etc., in addition to taking upon themselves a number of activities such as awareness generation, distributing ration, which have helped in fighting with the pandemic. These SHGs were till now seen as a mechanism to support women and their families from rural or disadvantaged backgrounds but now they are being envisaged as an important vehicle of economic recovery post Covid and the government has accordingly taken steps to strengthen them.

Self Help Group is a voluntary organization of enterprising people with a common goal, small and manageable, based on internal strength, aimed at making women socially and economically empowered. Its aim is to achieve economy of scale, and collective strength. The origin of micro-finance may be traced to Prof. Mohammed Yunus who started Grameen Bank in Chhittagong, Bangladesh in 1976. In India it was started in 1992 in Andhra Pradesh. Presently there are several SHGs working in India, notable amongst them being Kudumbshree in Kerala and SEWA in Gujarat. Although their main aim was to empower the vulnerable section of the society in rural as well as urban areas, by imparting life skills, livelihood, confidence, resourcefulness and a collective strength to women, their contribution in the present crisis has gone much beyond and has extended a much needed cushion effect to the most marginalized people by providing them means of livelihood and a sense of duty in tackling the Covid crisis. Approximately 690 lakh women members of around 63 lakh Self Help Groups (SHGs) across the country formed under the Deendayal Antyodaya Yojana- National Rural Livelihoods Mission (DAY-NRLM), Ministry of Rural Development, have emerged as community warriors by contributing in every possible way to contain the spread of COVID-19.[1] These foot soldiers have risen to the challenge and are contributing immensely by stitching masks, running community kitchens, fighting false information and ensuring door to door ration supply. In this battle for human survival, they are adapting rapidly to the new needs. With their resilient work, they are complimenting the over-burdened government machinery. In addition these are minimizing the negative impact of the pandemic such as job loss, loos of livelihood, and stress, providing a lifeline of engagement and hope much needed at this time, with a sense of contribution and self-worth.

While government formulates policies to boost the economy, SHGs may become an effective tool to revive the rural and urban economy with added benefits of multiplier effects of empowering women financially and socially. Therefore, it is imperative to pay attention to remove the structural barriers in order to leverage their full potential in recovery post Covid-19. This paper seeks to highlight the role women SHGs are playing in the present pandemic as well as provide suggestions on ways to utilize them in post Covid-19 rebuilding of the society, economy and the nation.

Objectives and Functioning of Self Help Group

The objectives of Self Help Group are development of leadership qualities, confidence building, increasing social awareness, improving the status of women in family and society, improvement of family welfare, functional literacy, awareness of legal rights, economic development, inculcating the habit of savings, increasing income, increasing assets, access to market choice of activities, and getting out of money lenders' clutches. The SHGs work in a democratic manner. The upper limit in the group is restricted to 20. One of the members is selected as an animator and two members are selected as representatives. The animator is selected for two years. The group members meet every week. They discuss about the group saving, rotation of funds, bank loan, repayment of loan, social and community action programs. The SHGs follow '*Panchsutras*' viz. conduct of regular group meetings, regular savings within the group, internal lending based on the demand of members, timely repayment of loan and maintenance of proper books of accounts.[2]

Financing of SHGs

Entrepreneurship through Self- Help group is promoted by the government of India and non-government organizations. The Micro,

Small and Medium Enterprises Development Act 2006 seeks to facilitate the development of entrepreneurship. Through Self Help Groups the endeavor has been to encourage women to contribute to family and community poverty reduction and their development. The following government programs support women workers with finance:

- MSE Cluster Development Program
- Credit Guarantee Fund Scheme for Micro and Small Enterprises
- Deendayal Antyodaya Yojana – National Rural Livelihoods Mission (DAY-NRLM), under Ministry of Rural Development. The programme aims to ensure that at least one woman member from each rural poor household (about 9 crore) is brought into the fold of women SHGs and their federations within a definite time frame. A Revolving Funds (RF) @ Rs.10,000-15,000 per SHG and Community Investment Support Fund (CISF) @ maximum of Rs.2,50,000 per SHG is provided to Self Help Groups (SHGs) and their Federations to take up self-employment for income generation.
- Deendayal Antyodaya Yojana – National Urban Livelihoods Mission (DAY-NULM) under Ministry of Housing and Urban Affairs. Under Social Mobilization and Institution Development (SM&ID) component, the mission envisages universal social mobilization of urban poor into Self-Help Groups (SHGs) and their Federations by bringing at least one member from each urban poor household, preferably a woman, under the SHG network.
- Under the Self-Employment Programme (SEP), interest subvention over and above 7 percent rate of interest is available to all SHGs accessing bank loans. An additional 3 percent interest subvention is also available to all women SHGs who repay their loan in time.[3]
- Through Self Help Group – Bank Linkage Programme (SHG-BLP), NABARD (National Bank for Agricultural and Rural Development) coopted many others as Self Help Promoting Institutions (SHPIs) including the rural financial institutions

(RRBs, DCCBs, PACS), Farmers' Clubs (FCs), SHG Federations, Individual Rural Volunteers (IRVs) etc. This savings led microfinance model has now become the largest coordinated financial inclusion programme in the world covering almost 100 million households in the country. With more than 84% of the groups being exclusively women groups, the programme has provided the much needed push to empowerment of women in the country.[4]

Role of SHGs in Changed Times of Covid-19

SHGs in India started to empower the rural poor women and to bring them out of poverty, however in these tough times of Covid-19 pandemics, this institution has turned into a huge support to the government. By being self-reliant they have not only reduced the burden from government but also have supplemented the official efforts to fight the pandemic in several ways. They are meeting shortfalls in masks, sanitizers and protective equipment, running community kitchens, fighting misinformation and even providing banking and financial solutions to far-flung communities.

> *"Women at the center of development has been an important story in South Asia. In these extraordinary times, when we are all united in our fight against the Covid 19 virus, these women's groups are playing a critical role."*
>
> **Junaid Ahmad**
>
> *World Bank country director in India*[5]

In Odisha, for instance, poor rural women who were once engaged in stitching school uniforms are sewing masks instead. Over the past couple of weeks, these women have produced more than 1 million cotton masks, helping equip police personnel and health workers, while earning something for themselves. More than 19 million masks have been produced by some 20,000 SHGs across 27 Indian states, in addition to over 100,000 liters of sanitizer and nearly 50,000 liters of hand wash. Since production is decentralized, these items have reached widely-dispersed populations without the need for complex logistics and transportation.[6]

In Uttar Pradesh Afsana Khan who heads an SHG of Chikankari artisans, started making masks of cotton. Later U.P. government collaborated with them and gave assignment to make handspun khadi masks. Besides the members of the SHG, many women with sewing machines at homes were also called upon to undertake the task, the fabric for which came from the Khadi and Village Industries Department. Ajay Kumar Singh, block development officer of Chinhat in Lucknow said that within three days since production of masks began, some 4,000 triple layer khadi masks have been made in the block he holds charge of. He estimated that across the eight blocks of Lucknow, this number would stand at 60,000. The khadi masks are moving through cooperatives, government departments and village pradhans.[7]

Fighting Hunger through Community Kitchens

The suspension of economic activities has sent a lot of people below poverty line and the daily wage earners struggle to make ends meet. In such a scenario, hunger has become a challenging issue. With huge numbers of informal workers losing their livelihoods during the lockdown and food supply chains getting disrupted in some areas, SHGs have set up over 10,000 community kitchens across the country to feed stranded workers, the poor, and the vulnerable. In Kerala, the Kudumbashree network, one of the country's earliest community platforms of women with 4.4 million members and several years of catering experience, were the government's natural choice to run a number of these kitchens. Given the massive nature of the challenge, these groups have dramatically ramped up their efforts and are now running 1,300 kitchens across the state, while also delivering food to those in quarantine and the bedridden.

In Jharkhand, where poverty is high, SHGs - being the closest to the ground - are helping district administrations identify pockets of hunger and starvation so efforts can be made to ameliorate them.[8]

Helping through Information Dissemination

Importantly, the SHGs are helping curb rumor and misinformation. The women are systematically using their vast network of WhatsApp groups to ward off chaos and confusion, providing critical support to the government in this hour of need. The devastating impact on migrant labor, where huge numbers of suddenly out-of-work families started walking back to their villages hundreds of miles away, shows how critical it is for authentic information to filter down to the grassroots. Women's groups are also disseminating Covid related messages among hard-to-reach populations. In Kerala, Kudumbashree is spearheading the government's Break the Chain campaign by raising awareness about hand hygiene and social distancing through mobile phones, posters and weekly meetings. In Bihar, one of India's poorest states, JEEViKA - the state's SHG platform – is spreading the word about handwashing, quarantine and self-isolation through leaflets, songs, videos and phone messages. JEEViKA has collected mobile numbers of more than 1,00,000 of community members and is using the Mobile Vaani platform to release voice messages on COVID-19 and is also addressing the community's queries through the same.

Women are also running help desks, and delivering food supplies to the elderly and the quarantined. In Jharkhand, where large numbers of people migrate to other states to work, they are running a dedicated helpline for returning migrants and other vulnerable families.[9]

Providing Banking and Pension Services

Since access to finance is critical for people to sustain themselves during the lockdown, SHG women who also work as banking correspondents have emerged as a vital resource. Deemed as an essential service, these *bank sakhis* have continued to provide doorstep banking services to far-flung communities, in addition to distributing pensions and enabling the most needy to access credits into their accounts through direct benefit transfers (DBT). Banks have given these women special orientation and provided them with financial incentives to enable them to continue to work during the lockdown.

"Across the country, women's SHGs have risen to this extraordinary challenge with immense courage and dedication," summed up Alka Upadhyay, Additional Secretary in India's Ministry of Rural Development, which manages the NRLM.

Ration Delivery

Their quick response to food insecurity and shortages in goods and services shows how this decentralized structure can be a vital resource in a time of crisis. The strength of India's rural women will continue to be essential in building back economic momentum after the most critical period is over.[10]

Members of two Kudumbshree units in Kainakary grama panchayat in Kuttanad have joined hands to come up with a floating supermarket, Thanima, to cater to hundreds of families affected by the lockdown, imposed following Covid-19, in a place surrounded by water. They have rented a boat and turned it into a floating store. The boat cruises the Pampa river every day offering consumers a new shopping experience with multi-brand products, including rice, locally produced vegetables, spices, egg, fruits, snacks, beverages, dried fish, nonfood items etc. The floating supermarket connects at least eight places in the area, including Patel Jetty, Malechira, Kochugovindan Jetty, Palli Jetty etc. Before starting from the Panchayat Kadavu, approximate time of the boat's arrival at respective boat jettis will be sent to mobile phones of members of neighbourhood groups, local ward members among others, which helps the people to come and buy commodities without waiting long.[11]

Social Distancing

SHG volunteers are playing their role in ensuring that people maintain social distancing in markets, PDS shops etc. In Tamil Nadu, two volunteers of SHGs are assigned to each PDS shop. They are provided gloves, masks and sanitizers and they ensure that people in the queue maintain adequate distance.

Rangolis for awareness

SHGs are using innovative communication and behaviour change tools to generate awareness and help containment of the COVID-19 infection. SHG women from UP SRLM 'Prerna' have used their creativity to make rangolis and mark lines and circles to re-emphasise the need for 'social distancing'. They have also been making wall paintings to spread key messages about COVID prevention in their communities.

Didi Helpline

The Didi helpline, a telephonic helpline initiated by Jharkhand SRLM, is open 24 hours to help migrant labourers by providing them verified information. It enables them to provide their data to state authorities to help evacuate them from different states, back to Jharkhand.[12]

Government Initiative to Promote SHGs

One of the major hurdles that the SHGs face in utilizing their full potential is lack of access to markets and the exposure to the urban customers' demands. To facilitate this access the Government of India has recently taken an initiative to display the SARAS collection on the government online procurement portal GeM (Government e-Marketplace). It is a unique initiative by the GeM, Deendayal Antyodaya Yojana-National Rural Livelihoods Mission (DAY-NRLM) and Ministry of Rural Development. The Saras Collection showcases daily utility products made by rural Self-Help Groups (SHGs) and aims to provide SHGs in rural areas with market access to Central and State Government buyers. The on-boarding of the SHGs has been initially piloted in the states of Bihar, Chhattisgarh, Jharkhand, Karnataka, Kerala, Himachal Pradesh, Maharashtra, Odisha, Rajasthan, Uttar Pradesh and West Bengal. SHGs from all the states and Union Territories (UTs) will be covered rapidly in the upcoming phases. The Saras Collection will provide SHGs with direct access to Government buyers which will do away with intermediaries in the supply chain, thus ensuring better prices for SHGs and spurring employment opportunities at the local level. The following mechanism will be followed:

- For Functionaries: They will be provided dashboards at the national, state, district and block level for real time information about the number of products uploaded, their value and volume of orders received and fulfilled.
- Government buyers: They will be sensitized through system generated messages/ alerts in the Marketplace about availability of SHG products on the portal.

GeM will collaborate with State functionaries to address the capacity building and training needs of SHGs and build up their competencies required for order packaging, catalogue management and logistics. GeM will develop online learning resources in vernacular content for SHGs with inputs and assistance from the NRLM and the State Rural Livelihoods Missions (SRLMs). For a seamless learning experience, GeM will conduct online webinars, develop videos, eBooks, manual and repository of FAQs.[13]

Providing the details of 1.76 lakh crore economic recovery stimulus package under the Pradhan Mantri Gareeb Kalyan Yojana the Union Finance Minister Nirmala Sitharaman stated that 7200 new SHGs have been opened since March 15, 2020. The limit of collateral free loan to SHGs has been doubled from Rs. 10 Lakh to Rs. 20 Lakh. State owned Indian Overseas Bank has launched a special scheme for SHGs to provide them loans to tide over the tough times. Under this special borrowing program, each SHG member is eligible to take loan upto Rs. 5000, and each SHG that has a history of having taken two loans from the Indian Overseas Bank, can take a loan of Rs. 01 lakh. No processing or pre-payment fee will be charged.[14]

Recently, in July 2020, the Uttar Pradesh government has initiated an exercise to merge self-help groups to form a bigger organizational structure, Community Level Federation (CLF), under the Centre's flagship scheme National Rural Economic Transformation Project (NRETP). A single CLF would be a registered body comprising at least 300 SHGs, and having at least 3,000 women, which would be engaged in manufacturing of saleable products. The Rural Development Department would initially provide support to CLFs so that they start with an initial capital, acting as a bank to disburse fund to SHGs with an interest rate of around 6%. In the initial phase, 15 SHGs would be merged to form a village organization. "About 15-20 village organisations will then be merged to form a CLF which would be a bigger structure to lend a fillip to the execution of NRETP.[15]

Suggestions to Unleash the SHG Potential

The challenges faced by SHGs include patriarchal mindset, lack of education, technological unawareness, inadequate infrastructure, finance limitation, lack of sufficient raw material, and market linkage. Therefore in order to utilize their full potential more capacity building programs need to be initiated to train the members in computer and soft skills, enable them in using digital space for connecting with raw material providers and distribution networks. Online training may be imparted to them about keeping records, dealing with banks on seeking loans, accounting and marketing their products on online platforms. In this context, e-Shakti program by NABARD launched in 2017 for digitization of SHGs is noteworthy. It was initiated to address certain concerns like improving the quality of book keeping of SHGs and to enable banks to take informed credit decisions about the group through a Management Information System (MIS).

Government, NGOs and corporates shall come forward to assist SHGs to improve their product quality to international standard, certification and branding may be done to enhance credibility. Women members must be seen as active participants rather than mere beneficiaries and their suggestions and opinion be sought while formulating policies regarding SHGs as they can bring out the ground level challenges and ways to ameliorate them. This will increase the effectivity of the schemes.

Conclusion

Sustaining their livelihoods through socially responsive contributions in promoting safe hygiene practices within their respective communities, these SHG women have been fighting the COVID 19 outbreak with utmost dedication and devotion. Through many similar responsible collective actions organized across the nation, marginalised and vulnerable women of these communities have played a significant role in the war against Coronavirus while being empowered both socially and economically.[16]

Afsana Khan, who was awarded by the state government for her entrepreneurial skills in 2017, says the masks are symbols of empowerment. "The men are at home without work while the women contribute to this very important task. This has made men look at the women with respect. It is the men who come to take the fabric and drop off the finished product at the facilitation centre. The look of relief and gratitude on their faces is visible. To earn Rs. 100-200 per day in these difficult times is a respite."[17]

The government has rightly realized the potential of SHGs in revival of economy and mitigating the social fallouts of the pandemic. It is reflected in the recent announcement by the Finance Minister of doubling the collateral free loans to women SHGs from Rs. 10 lakh to Rs. 20 Lakhs. Since these loans are neutral i.e. for both production and consumption purposes, these will give a boost to rural demand and consumption and will facilitate spending and investment both, the twin engine of economy. Since the NPA (Non-Performing Assets) percentage of SHGs is 4.5%, half than the normal NPA percentage in the Indian banking system[18], the need of the hour is that banks shall adopt a more liberalized approach in giving loans to the SHGs to boost the rural economy. Armed with technological upgradation, and financial and distributive network linkages, the women SHGs can emerge as a powerful tool to rebuild the economy, society and nation. They can act as a grass-root level catalyst of realizing the vision of *Atma Nirbhar Bharat* (self-reliant India).

References

1. NRLM Self Help Group network rises to the challenge of COVID-19 situation in the country, Press Information Bureau, Government of India, Ministry of Rural Development, 12-April-2020.
2. Micro Credit Innovation,. NABARD, https://www.nabard.org/content1.aspx?id=518&catid=8&mid=489.
3. Self Help Groups, Press Information Bureau, Government of India Ministry of Women and Child Development, information was given by the Minister of Women and Child Development, Smriti Zubin Irani, in a written reply in the Lok Sabha on 12-July-2019.
4. Micro Credit Innovation, NABARD, https://www.nabard.org/content1.aspx?id=518&catid=8&mid=489.
5. In India, women's self-help groups combat the COVID-19 (Coronavirus) pandemic, The World Bank Group, April 11, 2020, https://www.worldbank.org/en/news/feature/2020/04/11/women-self-help-groups-combat-covid19-coronavirus-pandemic-india
6. In India, women's self-help groups combat the COVID-19 (Coronavirus) pandemic, The World Bank Group, April 11, 2020 , https://www.worldbank.org/en/news/feature/2020/04/11/women-self-help-groups-combat-covid19-coronavirus-pandemic-india.

7. Awasthi Puja, Making a buck, waging a war: How women SHGs fight COVID-19 in UP, The Week, April 13, 2020.
8. In India, women's self-help groups combat the COVID-19 (Coronavirus) pandemic, The World Bank Group, April 11, 2020 , https://www.worldbank.org/en/news/feature/2020/04/11/women-self-help-groups-combat-covid19-coronavirus-pandemic-india
9. In India, women's self-help groups combat the COVID-19 (Coronavirus) pandemic, The World Bank Group, April 11, 2020 , https://www.worldbank.org/en/news/feature/2020/04/11/women-self-help-groups-combat-covid19-coronavirus-pandemic-india
10. In India, women's self-help groups combat the COVID-19 (Coronavirus) pandemic, The World Bank Group, April 11, 2020 , https://www.worldbank.org/en/news/feature/2020/04/11/women-self-help-groups-combat-covid19-coronavirus-pandemic-india
11. Paul Sam A., In Alappuzha, floating supermarket brings essentials to the doorstep of lockdown-affected, The Hindu, Allappuzha, April 05, 2020.
12. NRLM Self Help Group network rises to the challenge of COVID-19 situation in the country, Press Information Bureau, Government of India, Ministry of Rural Development, 12-April-2020.
13. Saras Collection, Drishti IAS, 05 May 2020, https://www.drishtiias.com/daily-updates/daily-news-analysis/saras-collection
14. Covid-19: Indian Overseas Bank launche special scheme for self help groups, The Indian Express, 27 April, 2020, Last Updated: 27th April 2020 02:34 PM, https://www.newindianexpress.com/business/2020/apr/27/covid 19-indian-overseas-bank-launches-special-scheme-for-self-help-groups-2135961.html
15. Shah Pankaj, SHG Clusters to widen jobs ambit for migrants, The Times of India, July 7, 2020, p.1.
16. NRLM Self Help Group network rises to the challenge of COVID-19 situation in the country, Press Information Bureau, Government of India, Ministry of Rural Development, 12-April-2020.
17. Awasthi Puja, Making a buck, waging a war: How women SHGs fight COVID-19 in UP, The Week, April 13, 2020.
18. Mishra Hari Hara, Self Help Group potential can boost rural production and consumption, The Economic Times, April 06, 2020.

6

Covid-19: Emanation, Emasculation and Emancipation- Demystifying Environmental Concerns

— *Dr. Shalini Pathak*

We belong to the 21st century, a century which exhibits progression, evolvement, improvement, development, breakthroughs, and aligns well with advanced technology. The commencement of 21st century *in toto* ushers a new era for mankind with convenience-oriented life and has also invited a stark contrast between human beings and environment. Besides the fact that we are associated to the most evolved generations, tremendous askew is observed in our environment. Today our Planet Earth is confronting gigantic environmental issues which not only possess infinite ability to devastate mankind, but also poses a threat even to its existence.

The environmental concerns like air pollution, water pollution, loss of biodiversity, excessive production of waste, climatic alterations, acidic rain, smog, depletion of ozone layer, emission of toxic gases, global warming, deforestation, urbanization, population explosion have catastrophic repercussions. The erratic pattern of human behavior is over-arching and is inclusive of multi-dimensional exploitation like over exhaustion of fossil fuel, over indulgence in the extraction of minerals, over consumption of natural resources, overbearing constructions, over population, over utilization of non-degradable products like plastic, overload of waste and destructing biodiversity. Without a doubt, COVID-19 is the direct repercussion of this over weening attitude of humans.

A look at the birthplace of this pandemic is sufficient to point out the interconnection of pandemics and human indicators. The disease made its first appearance in Wuhan of China, which is the capital city of Hubei province, and is an important commercial centre, divided by two rivers- Yangtze and Han. It is not only the largest city in Hubei province but also the most populated one in Central China. Does it indicate that a high pressure of population on land, and resultant change in land use, its adverse effect on biodiversity, reduced human-animal buffer, the heat effect and the clustered settlements leading to unhygienic conditions are conducive conditions for origin of an infectious disease? That the high population density makes it possible for an infection to spread faster takes only common sense to apprehend. The researchers have validated these points that the high frequency and the high morbidity rate of infectious diseases are deeply correlated with anthropogenic activities which adversely affect the Natural ecosystems. The paper presents a detailed analysis of these activities and their consequences on human health. It intends to generate a deeper understanding of the WHO's concept of "One Health" which propounds that the health of human beings, animals, and plants is interdependent, as all are the coexisting components of one ecosystem on the planet earth. To see human beings as separate entities from other living beings and even the non-living components of nature was the biggest mistake of human race which has been haunting it repeatedly in the form of infectious diseases, springing up frequently, and serving as a reminder to review the conquering attitude of humans. COVID-19 is the latest warning in that series and we can only ill afford to neglect it.

Comprehending Environment Conversions

The detached attitude adopted by us towards our environment has only compelled our environment to oscillate between depletion and augmentation, whether it is the depletion of ozone layer or augmentation of global warming, depletion of forests or augmentation of waste, depletion of biodiversity or augmentation of carbon dioxide in the air, our contribution towards keeping up the pace of depletion and augmentation process is whacking great. However, the acceleration witnessed an acute steep post-COVID 19. Undoubtedly, the impact of COVID-19 is enormous and significantly this impact can be visualized as the reversal of depletion and augmentation process wherein the human activity has witnessed a sharp deplete and environment a splendid augmentation. The relief brought by a cool breeze, the serenity of quietness due to ban on vehicular movement, the pleasing trill of birds, the heartening sight of wildlife roaming without fear and rivers becoming cleaner would remain etched in many a minds as a memorable glimpse of an environment that could have been if not for human intervention.

Air Pollution

Toxic air is one of the major environmental concerns, and is the oldest form of air pollution. Polluted air is not a recent phenomenon, in fact amongst all the environmental concerns, air pollution is the most deep- rooted therefore the implications of air pollution are not only drastically high but it also works as a catalyst to trigger other environmental concerns. It is better to say that air pollution is the foundation of all the existing environmental concerns, henceforth requires more attention. The outbreak of pandemic eventuated in the depletion of carbon dioxide emissions in the air, as a steep decline was observed in transportation and mobility process. Prohibition imposed on air travel, roadways travel, railways has been the most appropriate and prudent decision as it successfully contributed in the depletion process of carbon emissions.

A significant drop in the air pollution is apparently visualized which is directly proportional to the climatic change. According to the estimation of World Health Organization 80% of people residing in urban areas are exposed to depleted air quality which invites deadly health issues.[1] In fact in Beijing, the levels of toxicity in the air soared high and eventuated in a new form of diseases called the Beijing Cough. 65% of deaths in Asia and 25% of deaths in India are due to air pollution.[2]

The European Space Agency in its survey and research conducted from January 01 to March 11, 2020, has mentioned about a steep decline in the emissions of nitrous oxide from vehicles, power plants and industries in Italy.[3] Improvement in the air quality has also contributed in making the water more clean and clear and this magnified visibility and transparency of water is directly interlinked to the aquatic system which too has exhibited signs of improvement. In fact the healthier air quality is also indicative of the snow formation on hills and glacier formation. The entire system is so well interconnected that any sort of augmentation or depletion triggers a chain reaction effecting the entire system whether the atmosphere, lithosphere or the hydrosphere.

Deforestation

Another significant environmental concern is deforestation, which shares a direct pro rata relation with the emanation of COVID-19. The loss of forest land is a major concern, as half of the world's land has been converted to agricultural land, and deterioration of tropical forest is the most bewildering issue. It is important to comprehend the fact that forest is the living space and natural habitat of wildlife and animals. More clearance of forest apparently means demolition of the living space and dwellings of animals, which in turn indicates the need of new shelter and domain.

Since the forest habitat is shrinking at a fast pace it clearly indicates increased interaction between the wildlife and humans, sharing corresponding spaces and hunting for the same food. The major reason for the destruction of these forest and natural habitat of wildlife is the increased demand and commercial consumption of natural resources. This resource-oriented destruction eventuates in the unrestricted mobility of the wildlife which is symptomatic of transmission of animal to human diseases, often termed as zoonatic or zoonoses.[4]

Human intrusion into natural habitat and increasing proximity between humans and wildlife has also magnified the risk factor of transmission of diseases. The frequency of deforestation after crossing the saturation point amplifies the intensity of transmission of disease irrespective of the fact whether the humans are in contact with the wildlife. A study conducted by the School of Earth Energy and Environmental Sciences has suggested that the demolition of forests has increased the transmission of zoonotic diseases and the basic reason for the emanation of COVID-19 is deforestation.

According to epidemiologists, when the natural habitat remains intact and undisturbed by human interference and activities these viruses keep circulating in mild forms in animals, but when human destruction of natural habitat commences, it disrupts the entire equilibrium and the viruses come in contact with the humans which eventuates in development of several bacterial and viral infections. It is estimated that 80,000 acre of tropical forests is being destroyed per day and this ruination becomes more vicious and threatening when we observe the end result of deforestation which is 15% of the world's greenhouse gas emissions,[5] making the earth warmer and creating more conducive temperatures for pathogens to survive and thrive.

Imbalances in Biodiversity

The perpetuation of our environment is based on the fundamentals of biodiversity, a factor which works as a catalyst for the preservation and conservation of our environment. The importance of biological diversity can be well comprehended from the fact that it blankets every species existing on this earth, whether it is animals, birds, aquatic life, micro-organism or plants. All the species form a constitutive part of the ecosystem. However, continuous human interference has not only disrupted biodiversity but has also impeded the growth of biodiversity and has resulted in triggering the development of viruses and diseases. David Quammen in his book *Spillover: Animal Infections and the Next Pandemic* has mentioned, "We cut the trees, we kill the animals or cage them and then send them to markets. We disrupt the ecosystems, and we shake viruses loose from their natural hosts. When that happens, they need a new host. Often we are it."[6] It is important to comprehend the fact that the entire system works on balance, if the wildlife equilibrium witnesses human trespass then human life too will be interfered and disrupted by the animals.

Tackling Contaminated Waste

United Nations Environment Programme is one of the most pivotal and phenomenal organizations working for the advancement of the environment cause. The impact of COVID-19 has been on every aspect of life, but the major problem which crops up here is the fact that in order to tackle the entire situation waste material generated in large amounts is a growing concern now. The pattern in which the unrestricted hazardous waste is supplementing, it's undoubtedly symptomatic of severe imminent ramifications in an unseemly manner.

In such sort of crisis situation, several places like hospitals, market places, garbage zones become a repository of toxic and contaminated waste which requires instantaneous foolproof disposable system. It is this infallible system of discarding waste which if conducted methodically and systematically axes down the multiplied effect of hazardous waste, but if mishandled would enhance the multiplication. UNEP has been supremely responsive as far as the entire waste management programme is concerned. An International environmental agreement on the management and disposal of hazardous waste has been formulated at the Basel Convention with the clear objective of protecting and securing environment and mankind from the ill-effects and impact of toxic waste.[7]

It is estimated that average person produces 4.3 pounds of waste per day, with America single-handedly generating 20 million tons of waste every year. The waste contribution is significantly high which in turn ends up in the production of methane gas, which is not only toxic and hazardous for the environment but it is one of the most dangerous greenhouse gas, owing to its potential of amplifying global warming.[8]

Change in Climate

Climate is another major issue as far as COVID-19 is concerned. Today the climate has witnessed a significant change no matter whether it's a vertical drop or a horizontal drop, the pace at which the skies have transformed from grey to white is astonishing. Undoubtedly the impact of COVID-19 on human lives is devastating but we cannot ignore the fact that its impact on our environment is constructive and affirmative. The transformation of pollution scale from grey to white has been significant and apparent.

With tourism, travel and aviation sector coming to a halt, 2% of global emissions have reduced, at least 10 million metric tons less carbon dioxide is emitted from aviation.[9] According to Europe's Euro Control Agency about 80% of international flight activity has been cut back. With no traffic in the air and also on roads, the demand and consumption of oil and crude oil has declined drastically. Reduction in the air pollution also contributed to reduction in the noise pollution. The muted atmosphere has given way to the birds chirping and has also paced up the healing process of the environment.

It is important to comprehend the nature of COVID-19, which directly attacks our respiratory system, as the symptoms of COVID-19 is all about sneezing, cough, cold and fever. All these symptoms are directly associated to our lungs and respiration system. Weak lungs, asthma, chronic lung condition are other contributory factors which push the vulnerability boundary of COVID-19. It is at this point when the inhalation and exhalation process becomes important, the better the air quality, healthier is the state of lungs and which in turn shrinks the impact of COVID-19.

Assessment

History has seen outbreak of several pandemics, whether it's the ancient, medieval or modern times, and every pandemic not only brought with itself portents of disaster, but have also severely changed the course of time, bringing in several historical, political, economic and religious alterations. COVID-19 is an admonition to human beings for their disoriented conduct towards the environment. Calmness and serenity is the nature of Nature, however, in the present scenario the agony of nature is apparent which has exposed mankind to the zenith of vulnerability, with strong revelations, diminishing the hitherto thick demarcation line of the developed, developing and underdeveloped nations.

COVID-19 is like a Sword of Damocles, which requires global participation and attention, irrespective of the development stage of nations, indubitably the concern is enveloping the whole world.

COVID-19 is completely free from the filtration process and when the dimension of no filters comes in, the concept of sparing diminishes altogether. The long term impassivity and torpid state of mind has brought mankind on the verge of collapse. It is the period of comprehending the importance of 'R', which stands for realization and respite, with realization a necessity for human beings and respite for the environment.

Innovation was and is a necessity, but we humans rigorously performed innovation without respecting the limitations of innovations and ignoring the limitless Mother Nature. It was at this critical juncture when Mother Nature decided to teach humans a few lessons, with powerful telltales. Nature's format for cleaning the environment, centuries ago was visualized more in the form of droughts, famines, volcanic eruption, floods or any other form of natural calamity, but with the increased human interference, the disposition, complexion and format of these natural calamities have also witnessed a drastic change, and is now visualized in the outbreak of threatening diseases, epidemics, pandemics as in the form of Swine Flu, Influenza, Zika, Ebola and Corona virus, with results being the same, loss of mankind.

The situation of COVID-19 has transformed the entire world into a circle. To maintain the concept of social distancing, circles have been made, within which human beings are captured. There is no doubt that nature's agony is expressed in the form of excruciatingly painful COVID-19. The convenience-oriented lifestyle and the thick commercial consumption has so firmly clutched our minds that we are bereft of our moral responsibilities and insight. It is definitely not prudent to say that environment is above mankind and life of human beings, but the pattern in which the eroded environment is replenishing itself also poses an open question to the human behavior towards Nature. It is important to strike a balance between humans and environment in order to alter and axe down the negative impact of COVID-19. Undoubtedly the emanation of COVID-19 on one hand has emasculated the power and authority enjoyed by the humans for increasing the exploitation process and on the other hand it has hastened the emancipation process of environment by rendering it a much needed respite.

The admonishing signs delivered by Mother Nature have said it all that however evolved and intellectual species we become when it comes to resilient and tranquil nature, we are not even a speck of dust. However advanced and technologically upgraded we become, we cannot blink our eyes to the fact that neither we have the ability to bring another planet for human existence nor do we possess the capability to outweigh Mother Nature and her verdict. COVID-19 is actually the transfer of power which hitherto vested in the hands of humans, but today the paradigm shift is obvious.

References

1. https://en.wikipedia.org/wiki/Impact_of_the_COVID-19_pandemic_on_the_environment.
2. Renewable Resources Coalition, "Top 17 Environmental Problems", last updated: December 4, 2016.
   https://www.renewableresourcescoalition.org/top-environmental-problems/
3. Rinkesh, "Air Pollution Facts", Conserve Energy Future, accessed on 12 June 2020. https://www.conserve-energy-future.com/various-air-pollution- facts.php
4. World Economic Forum, "Forest loss could make diseases like COVID-19 more likely, according to study", 15 Apr 2020. https://www.weforum.org/agenda/2020/04/forest-loss-diseases-covid19-coronavirus-deforestation-health/
5. Padma T.V., "Deforestation and disease: How natural habitat destruction can fuel zoonotic diseases", Mongabay, 1 April 2020. https://india.mongabay.com/2020/04/deforestation-and-disease-how-natural-habitat-destruction-can-fuel-zoonotic-diseases/
6. Renewable Resources Coalition, "Top 17 Environmental Problems", last updated: December 4, 2016. https://www.renewableresourcescoalition.org/top-environmental-problems/
7. Vidal John, 'Tip of the iceberg': is our destruction of nature responsible for Covid-19?, The Guardian, Wed 18 Mar 2020 06.00 GMT.
   https://www.theguardian.com/environment/2020/mar/18/tip-of-the-iceberg-is-our-destruction-of-nature-responsible-for-covid-19-aoe
8. Renewable Resources Coalition, "Top 17 Environmental Problems", last updated: December 4, 2016. https://www.renewableresourcescoalition.org/top-environmental-problems/
9. Lombrana Laura Millan & Warren Hayley, "A Pandemic That Cleared Skies and Halted Cities Isn't Slowing Global Warming", Bloomberg Green, May 8, 2020, https://www.bloomberg.com/graphics/2020-how-coronavirus-impacts-climate-change/

7

Anxiety, Stress and Coping Strategies in Pandemics

— *Dr. Kumkum Singh*

Survival takes winning over a lot of adverse conditions. All the living creatures including human beings have an innate instinct to survive. The human race has evolved fighting with and conquering many existential challenges, be it natural disasters, weather, diseases or in more modern times the socio-economic and cultural pressures. When faced with an adversity, our instant reaction is of stress, anxiety and fighting spirit. Stress is a natural reaction which prepares our body to react fast and appropriately in a dangerous situation. According to Will Yacowicz, "When your brain detects a stressor, your hypothalamus releases the hormone cortisol, which then jumps into your blood stream and locks into receptors in your tissues and organs. Your blood sugar goes up, adrenaline raises your heart rate, and oxygen fills your muscles. Your body readies itself for a threat, the evolutionary reaction commonly known as "fight or flight."[1] However when there is no scope for any of these physical actions, the stress results in anxiety and fear of the unknown, harming our emotional well-being, which if prolonged may reflect in our physical illness also.

Though human existence has been punctuated with diseases and pandemics, COVID-19 has presented an unprecedented situation for most of us. Spanish Flu 1918 and other pandemics are only alive in our imagination through books and pictures but no actual experience of a pandemic had till now been inflicted upon our generation. Also other pandemics such as AIDS, Ebola, Malaria though prevalent, had not brought such disruption in our lives so as to bring everything to a standstill in the entire world. It has brought along with it the fear of human in humans themselves. The erstwhile established norms in every field have been flung into the dustbin by the invisible virus and no amount of scientific knowledge has yet come to our rescue. The feeling of helplessness in the wake of a microscopic entity is overwhelming. No sophisticated weapons, no shelters, no technology can afford us protection when humans themselves have been turned into potential threat. This knowledge of being dangerously vulnerable has raised anxiety level in people for their own safety and that of their loved ones. Suspension of economic activities have raised the fear of survival and lockdowns have enhanced feeling of loneliness across the human population. However, various organisations have come forward to issue advice and ways to cope with the pandemic induced stress. This paper would delve deep into the psychological factors behind stress and suggest ways to overcome it, reinstating hope and faith in the survival capability of human beings.

Fear Paramount

Coronavirus Disease 2019 (COVID-19) has been heralded as the invisible enemy, the angel of death, a relentless and soulless invader that has infected the global psyche with fear and the bodies of our most vulnerable citizens and the broader populace with a potentially lethal illness. In many communities, virtually every aspect of daily life has been turned topsy-turvy, from how people earn their livelihood, socialize, and recreate to worries about financial ruin. People keep their distance from one another, and live in fear, not knowing what challenges and perils the day or next days will bring, and if they or a loved one will survive the viral onslaught.[2]

Like other calamities COVID-19 is also likely to trigger adverse psychological reactions that encompass anxiety, acute stress, addictive behaviors, and posttraumatic stress symptoms, alongside increased suicidality, self-blame, and major depression. At the core of all these conditions lies elements of one of the most basic and primal human emotions - fear. In the case of COVID-19, it is inextricably tied to feelings of helplessness and the loss of a fundamental sense of safety, security, financial stability, and the ability to envision a brighter future. Fear of infection in the presence of others, of contact with contaminated surfaces, and of passing too close to another human being evokes an increasingly familiar shudder of mistrust of others, avoidance, and withdrawal from everyday activities, thereby shrinking our worlds and constraining opportunities for essential human contact and social support, which are vitally necessary for adaptive functioning. Isolation, a signature of the COVID-19 epidemic, places unique and severe strains on the ability to maintain a resilient posture, in contrast with natural disasters in which community members join together, physically and socially, with common purpose and energy to help others as the crisis unfolds and later rebuild what was destroyed.[3] Thus the unique feature of COVID-19 in terms of imposing isolation has enhanced the risk of emotional turmoil manifold. The vulnerable sections such as children, elderlies, differently abled may be more at the receiving end of the psychological effects of this pandemic. Thus the need is to understand the symptoms first in order to identify the requirement of early intervention.

Vulnerability for Increased Stress Level during the Pandemic

Change in our psychological state due to stress manifests itself in various forms. For ensuring our own well-being as well as of others around us, observation and identification of these symptoms can be very useful. Stress during an infectious disease outbreak can sometimes cause the following:

- Fear and worry about your own health and the health of your loved ones, your financial situation or job, or loss of support services you rely on.
- Changes in sleep or eating patterns.
- Difficulty sleeping or concentrating.
- Worsening of chronic health problems.
- Worsening of mental health conditions.
- Increased use of tobacco, and/or alcohol and other substances.[4]

Certain groups of people are more vulnerable to increased stress during a pandemic. These may include, people who are at higher risk for severe illness from COVID-19 (for example, older people and people with underlying health conditions), children and teens, people caring for family members or loved ones, frontline workers such as health care providers and first responders, retail clerks, and others, essential workers who work in the food industry, people with existing mental health conditions, people who use substances or have a substance use disorder, people who have lost their jobs, had their work hours reduced, or had other major changes to their employment, people who have disabilities or developmental delay, people who are socially isolated from others, including people who live alone, and people in rural or frontier areas, people in some racial and ethnic minority groups, people who do not have access to information in their primary language, people experiencing homelessness, people who live in congregate (group) settings[5] or residents of high infection incidence areas. Infact research suggests that women have also been facing more stress due to everyone being present at home because of lockdown which has increased their burden of care as well as instances of domestic violence and sexual exploitation.

Even among patients with common flu symptoms, stress and fear due to the similarity of the conditions can generate mental distress and worsen psychiatric symptoms. Despite the fact that the rate of confirmed vs. suspected cases of COVID-19 is relatively low and that the majority of cases are considered asymptomatic or mild, as well as that the disease has a relatively low mortality rate, the psychiatric implications can be significantly high, overloading emergency services and the health system as a whole.[6]

Ways to Reduce Stress

Stress building up in individuals is not only harmful for them but also for the entire society and humanity at large. It brings frustration, fatigue, and behavorial changes either excessive aggression or complete withdrawal. World Health Organisation has released a guide on how to cope with mental stress, titled, 'Doing What Matters in Times of Stress' which is an easy to understand and relate, illustrated guide and begins with identifying self emotions, the causes of sadness or stress and gradually "unhooking" ourselves with those negative thoughts.[7] Importance of values in replacing negative thoughts with the positive ones has been reiterated. It states that the crucial step to ensure well- being is to be kind to ourselves and to those around us. In dealing with the stress related to a pandemic, there are three components involved: Individual, the society and the official apparatus.

At individual level, taking care of one's health without getting overly worried is essential. For that the Centre for Disease Prevention and Control suggests the following:

- Know what to do if you are sick and are concerned about COVID-19. Contact a health professional before you start any self-treatment for COVID-19.
- Know where and how to get treatment and other support services and resources, including counseling or therapy (in person or through telehealth services).
- Take care of your emotional health. Taking care of your emotional health will help you think clearly and react to the urgent needs to protect yourself and your family.
- Take breaks from watching, reading, or listening to news stories, including those on social media. Hearing about the pandemic repeatedly can be upsetting.
- Take care of your body.
    - Take deep breaths, stretch, or meditate.
    - Try to eat healthy, well-balanced meals.
    - Exercise regularly.
    - Get plenty of sleep.
    - Avoid excessive alcohol use and drugs.
- Make time to unwind. Try to do some other activities you enjoy.
- Connect with others. Talk with people you trust about your concerns and how you are feeling.
- Connect with your community- or faith-based organizations. While social distancing measures are in place, consider connecting online, through social media, or by phone or mail.[8]

In the world flooded with social media news, anxiety is natural when one keeps listening to the rising numbers of infection, therefore it is advisable to get information only from the authentic sources and that too at a particular time of the day, to avoid confusion and overloading of mind. Art Markman, a professor of psychology and marketing at the University of Texas at Austin, wrote about the emotional mechanics of stress, "you need to work at identifying your issues and "break the cycle of rumination—the pattern of negative thoughts that accompanies, and worsens, stress." He says stress is perpetuated by negativity. If you find yourself in a negative cycle, try to focus on positive aspects of your life. Displacing negative thoughts with positive ones can help "you engage your approach motivational system rather than the avoidance system and open yourself up to more experiences of joy and satisfaction."[9]

Along with caring for self, comes caring for family and community members. We need to understand that pandemic disrupts the normal way of life and vulnerable segments such as children, elderly and differently able people react differently to these changes and therefore require deep psychological understanding and emotional support. In such situations children may seek more attachment and become demanding on the parents. WHO suggests finding positive ways to express their feelings of fear and sadness, such as painting, drawing, poems, playing and creating a routine for them along with increasing communication within the family. For elderlies, it is useful to provide them information in a clear way through pictures or in writing, and repeat patently if necessary, in addition to helping them maintain a hygiene routine.

Social stigma attached to a disease or pandemic is a big reason of stress in those affected or victims of unjust social branding. The society as a whole needs to be sympathetic and not stigmatizing since the affected ones have not done anything wrong. In its message to the general populace during the pandemic the World Health Organisation has emphasized on the need for understanding and support. Since pandemics affect people from a vast geographical area without distinction of race, religion, caste, gender or socio-economic status, it is wrong to attach the infection to any particular group. Also caution must be exercised in the use of terminology while referring to infected people. Rather than calling them, 'Covid Cases', or 'Victims', it is better to call them 'people who are being treated for Covid-19' or 'people who have recovered from Covid-19' in order to avoid attaching an identity to them related to the disease, which may trigger psychological impacts.[10]

Providing psychological first aid is an essential care component for populations that have been victims of emergencies and disasters, but there are no universal protocols or guidelines for the most effective psychosocial support practices. Although some reports on local mental health care strategies have been published, more comprehensive emergency guidelines for such scenarios are unknown, since previous evidence refers only to specific situations. Specifically for this new COVID-19 scenario, Xiang et al., suggest that three main factors should be considered when developing mental health strategies:

(1) Multidisciplinary mental health teams (including psychiatrists, psychiatric nurses, clinical psychologists and other mental health professionals);

(2) Clear communication involving regular, accurate updates on the COVID-19 outbreak; and

(3) Establishing safe psychological counseling services (for example, via electronic devices or apps).[11]

Importance of Research based Public Policies

Since government policies affect the socio-economic state of the people and hence indirectly their emotional well-being, it is extremely necessary to implement public mental health policies in conjunction with epidemic and pandemic response strategies before, during and after the event. Mental health professionals, such as psychologists, psychiatrists and social workers, must be on the front line and play a leading role in emergency planning and management teams. Assistance protocols, such as those used in disaster situations, should cover areas relevant to the individual and collective mental health of the population. Recently, the WHO and the U.S. Center for Disease Control and Prevention published a series of psychosocial and mental health recommendations. This is in line with longitudinal data from the WHO demonstrating that psychological factors are directly related to the main causes of morbidity and mortality in the world. Thus, increased investment in research and strategic actions for mental health in parallel with infectious outbreaks is urgently needed worldwide.[12]

To inform management of COVID-19, it is vital to understand the socio-economic effect of the policies used to manage the pandemic, which will inevitably have serious effects on mental health by increasing unemployment, financial insecurity, and poverty. Involvement of people with lived experience and rapid qualitative research with diverse people and communities will help to identify ways in which this negative effect might be alleviated. Achieving the right balance between infection control and mitigation of these negative socioeconomic effects must be considered.[13]

Conclusion

The Covid crisis has added to the already strained human mind due to the modern life styles and nuclear existence, coupled with the pressure to perform in a highly competitive world with limited resources. Due to the prescribed social distancing rules to avoid infection, the usual links of socio-emotional support have been broken. The problems related to physical well- being and associated effects of lockdown and economic derailment have started to manifest in increased depression. However, during adversity human beings have a capacity to harness the inner strength, reenergize themselves and find out a way to deal with the situation. It is a tough time for the entire humanity and therefore also a time to support each other not only in material terms but also on the emotional front. By slowing us down the pandemic has provided us an opportunity to revive our connection with ourselves, our family members, friends, community and the environment. Recognition of the need for communication and help is the first step towards well-being. Thus focus on the silver lining at the end of the cloud rather than the dark cloud itself. Combined efforts by individuals, communities, religious organisations, NGOs, multilateral organisations and mental health care professionals will sail us through collectively. In the words of His Holiness The Dalai Lama, it is time to reinforce the feeling of being "one human family" which will help in tiding over the feelings of loneliness, and helplessness. As one community, having faith in our own capabilities to rebuild and rejuvenate ourselves is the key to avoid stress and keep working towards the betterment. As Prem Jagyasi said, "During Lockdown, we are surely locked but not down. Stay inspired". Yoga, meditation, and pranayam are a good way to establish harmony within inner elements and becoming calm, looking at the present situation with the eternal knowledge that everything is impermanent and shall change.

References

1. Yacowicz Will, 'How to Reduce Stress by Learning the Science Behind What's Causing It', Inc, accessed on 30 June 2020, 16.34 IST, https://www.inc.com/will-yakowicz/how-to-leverage-science-of-stress-to-your-advantage.html#:~:text=When%20your%20brain%20detects%20a,and%20oxygen%20fills%20your%20muscles.
2. Polizzi, C., Lynn, S.J., Perry, A. (2020), Stress and Coping in the Time of COVID-19: Pathways to Resilience and Recovery, Clinical Neuropsychiatry, 17 (2), pp. 59-62, https://doi.org/10.36131/ CN20200204.
3. Polizzi, C., Lynn, S.J., Perry, A. (2020), Stress and Coping in the Time of COVID-19: Pathways to Resilience and Recovery, Clinical Neuropsychiatry, 17 (2), pp. 59-62, https://doi.org/10.36131/ CN20200204.
4. Coping with Stress, Centres for Disease Control and Prevention, Updated June 12, 2020.
5. Coping with Stress, Centres for Disease Control and Prevention, Updated June 12, 2020.
6. Ornell, Felipe, Schuch, Jaqueline B., Sordi, Anne O., & Kessler, Felix Henrique Paim. (2020). "Pandemic fear" and COVID-19: mental health burden and strategies. *Brazilian Journal of Psychiatry*, *42*(3), pp. 232-235. Epub April 03, 2020.https://doi.org/10.1590/1516-4446-2020-0008
7. 'Doing what matters in times of stress', World Health Organisation, 29 April, 2020, https://www.who.int/publications/i/item/9789240003927
8. Coping with Stress, Centres for Disease Control and Prevention, Updated June 12, 2020.
9. Yacowicz Will, 'How to Reduce Stress by Learning the Science Behind What's Causing It', Inc, accessed on 30 June 2020, 16.34 IST, https://www.inc.com/will-yakowicz/how-to-leverage-science-of-stress-to-your-advantage.html#:~:text=When%20your%20brain%20detects%20a,and%20oxygen%20fills%20your%20muscles.

10. Mental health and psychosocial considerations during the COVID-19 outbreak, WHO, 18 March 2020, https://apps.who.int/iris/bitstream/handle/10665/331490/WHO-2019-nCoV-MentalHealth-2020.1-eng.pdf
11. Ornell, Felipe, Schuch, Jaqueline B., Sordi, Anne O., & Kessler, Felix Henrique Paim. (2020). "Pandemic fear" and COVID-19: mental health burden and strategies. *Brazilian Journal of Psychiatry*, *42*(3), pp. 232-235. Epub April 03, 2020.https://doi.org/10.1590/1516-4446-2020-0008
12. Ornell, Felipe, Schuch, Jaqueline B., Sordi, Anne O., & Kessler, Felix Henrique Paim. (2020). "Pandemic fear" and COVID-19: mental health burden and strategies. *Brazilian Journal of Psychiatry*, *42*(3), pp. 232-235. Epub April 03, 2020.https://doi.org/10.1590/1516-4446-2020-0008
13. Prof. Emily AHolmes PhD, Prof. Rory CO'Connor PhD, *Prof. V Hugh Perry PhD, ProfIreneTracey PhD, [g]Prof. Simon Wessely MD, [i]Prof. Louise Arseneault PhD, [i]Prof. Clive Ballard PhD, [k]Prof. Helen Christensen PhD, [l]Prof. Roxane Cohen Silver PhD, [m]ProfIan Everall PhD, [i]Prof. Tamsin Ford PhD, [n]Prof. Ann John PhD, [p]Thomas Kabir PhD, [q]Kate King BSc [r]Prof Ira Madan MD [s]Prof Susan Michie PhD [e]Prof. Andrew KPrzybylski PhD, Prof. Roz Shafran PhD, [f]...Prof. Ed Bullmore PhD., 'Multidisciplinary research priorities for the COVID-19 pandemic: a call for action for mental health science', The Lancet, Psychiatry, Volume 7, Issue 6, June 2020, pp. 547- 560.

8

Unlocking COVID 19: Metamorphosing Society, Tradition, and Fine Arts

— Dr. Subhra Rajput

> *"The pandemic travelled through the air as if on wings, it burned through cities like fire."*[1]

The above lines best describe the situation the coronavirus disease (COVID-19) induced pandemic has brought with it. Since its first outbreak on 31st December 2019 in Wuhan, China, it has engaged the whole world into a relentless fight against it. The situation is even more perilous when one knows world is having no cure for it. Five months into the worst pandemic in a generation that has shutdown nation and forced the humanity indoors, there is no definite end in sight. Sars-CoV-2 infection has ripped its way through the globe and there is only one feasible option- large scale social distancing that requires a fundamental rethink of the ways in which we socialize, work and function in society.

When our Prime Minister Narendra Modi announced a 21 day national lockdown on March 24, 2020 to combat the coronavirus disease (COVID-19) epidemic, half a million people in the world were infected, 20,000 people had died, and the virus was rampaging through nations. Epidemiologists warned of alarming deaths and hospitalization without a vaccine and in the grip of the panic, world leaders adopted the Wuhan model of locking down citizens to combat the epidemic. India followed suit with Modi assuring the nation that the social distancing was the only way to counter the virus and the lockdown would break the chain of infection. With precaution as its only cure, over last few months life has been put under the lockdown; it has come to a standstill and 'stay home, stay safe' has become a new maxim. Scientists and medical experts are of strong opinion that the practice of ensuring a minimum distance of 6 feet between two people can help control the infection and has helped save tens and thousands of lives worldwide. According to Per Block, (the lead author of the study and the researcher at University of Oxford's Leverhulme Centre for Demographic Science and Department of Sociology) "our models demonstrate that while social distancing measures clearly do flatten the curve,"[2] it is necessary to split up people into smaller, insulated clusters of population to minimize the infection and hence slowing down the epidemic. Block further adds, "we can make judgements on which of our contacts are long range ties that would be avoided or if necessary for work, should be treated with utmost care. People that live far away, people that don't know any of our other contact, or people that we have not seen in a longer time-these are the contacts that carry the biggest risk."[3]

While masks, temperature checks and hand sanitizers have become prevalent, experts and authorities are looking at social distancing strategies as a new option than sweeping shutdowns that cripple national economies, batter income and can drive millions into poverty. Social distancing can play a pivotal role for living everyday life, whether it is for school children, essential workers, office people, meeting friends or going out. However, the idea of distance is a luxury in a poor country like ours with the second largest population in the world with large household sizes with many people often crammed into a single room. "Learning to live cautiously with the virus is the only pragmatic strategy…….with improved knowledge of the epidemic, returning to 'new normal' with adequate protection for the vulnerable, precautions of distancing and hygiene is the most optimum strategy,"[4] for now. There is extreme fear and panic among the people, as the coronavirus ranges across the world, the most rigorously and consciously prepared planning seems failing. While we are far from overcoming the pandemic at this stage, society at large is skeptical, petrified of contracting the infection. There is another side of the apprehension among people to start a new normal as there is also a stigma associated with the disease as the world learns more about the disease every day. There is now greater information, date and evidence to assess the lockdown strategy and chart a new one.

"To exit the lockdown or not- that is the question," lines from William Shakespeare play, best describe the Nation's dilemma. Unlike prince Hamlet this is not a question of one's own life but a billion other lives. It is critical to make decision on sound facts and evidence, not fear or hope.[5] But the question still looming large on the society and its people is from where they can begin or start anew. "Letting people interact in some manner is also crucial from a mental health perspective for prolonged social distancing is likely to lead to mental health outcomes, especially for those who do not have a robust support system and are struggling through this process alone," said Dr. Samir Parikh, Director, Department of Mental Health and Behavioral Sciences, Fords Healthcare. Thus, the unprecedented crisis that we currently face with covid-19 is, how to coexist with a virus? "How do life, work and play go on when a highly infective and potentially fatal disease is still," spreading its tentacles. "It is unlikely that there will be a tipping point, a safe after date beyond which virus will not pose a threat to humanity. And finally, when a vaccine is discovered it will be sometime before everyone in the world has been inoculated.... Yet life and work (even play) cannot wait...."[6] While shops and 'direct to consumer business' are slowly opening in India with significant restrictions as an experiment as a lead to the opening of other essentials like educational institutes, offices, businesses and other employments, one must be prepared to face significant restrictions on what you can and can't do. And where you can or cannot go. Obviously in such apprehensive times huge and large religious gatherings, recreational events, mammoth crowd for theatre and stage are out for now. Songs, premiers, and stage shows will be the very last thing on anybody's list of what is safe. The crisis is going to accelerate a trend that has gained strength in recent years, technology, and digitalization. It is no less than a miracle that within fortnight, technology suddenly become acceptable- even mandatory. From business conferences to webinars, online classes to our daily basic needs, from entertainment to new releases on the web, technology has taken over the world suddenly.

Few months back if somebody would have suggested to a religiously fervent country such as India, to have a digital *darshan* of the God, it's rituals and ceremonies or suggested digital Music summit to a crowd loving singer or a fan dancing in frenzy during the live performance of its favorite singer or the virtual world can be the stage for 75 global artists for digital performance or film loving crazy nation competing for the first day first show tickets, going far enough to trade it in black that the new film is to be released on the digital platforms would have suddenly and certainly raised brow or laughed on its absurdity. But things and times like that are here to stay. Theatre and musical performances will have to move online, and we will see significant innovations in the space, thanks to virtual reality and augmented reality. Fear of coronavirus disease will restrict our movements and interactions which will lead to improvisation and metamorphosing of society, tradition, and fine arts as it was not seen in the past hundreds of years.

Covid-19 is an unexpected event for all the followers of different religions and affiliations which has equally affected the religious practices across the globe. There is a little hope for revival of religious places till the fear of coronavirus persist. "Never in my lifetime I have seen lanes leading to temples in Mathura and Vrindavan lying so barren", says veteran of Brig literature, 85 year old Padma Shri awardee, Mohan Swaroop Bhatia.[7] With the cancellation of the worship services of various faiths, closure of Sunday school and mass, Friday prayers in mosques, temples and *gurudwaras* as well as the cancellation of pilgrimages observances and festivals, religion is set to discover itself anew. "The most dramatic result in religion has been the exceedingly quick shift of religious service from in person to online worship."[8] Religious places are adopting online technologies to stay connected with their devotees by webcasting *aartis, darshans* and others rituals. For the first time ever, the biggest celebration in Madurai, Chithirai Festival, a simple celestial union took place, that was streamed online. "We are under complete lockdown, but we're trying to stay connected with devotees who keep calling us for performing pujas inside the temple like before. We just tell them to wait for some more time. They can go online to our Facebook page where evening *Aarti* is webcast, said Mahant Divya Giri, head priest of Mankameshwar temple."[9] Not only temples but Islamic Centers are also live streaming evening *Taraweeh* (prayer), Churches are live streaming Sunday Mass and this year Good Friday and Easter (holy week) services were broadcast online.

Live music shows are facing crisis as multiple big tickets events across Mumbai, New Delhi, Bangalore, and Chennai were called off or postponed. "Some of the cancelled or postponed events in Live Music so far include: Road to Ultra shows in Delhi and Hyderabad.... Khalid's tour stops in Mumbai and Bengaluru. A few festivals, including BUDX in Mumbai and the hip hop focused Bira 91 April Fool's Fest in Delhi were pushed even before they were announced, sources tell Billboard."[10] With concerts cancelled, musicians and bands are reaching out to the public, and even gaining newer audience, through online gigs. Oorli band were having a packed schedule for performances when outbreak happened. Forced to cancel it, they have been performing live every night to the audience across the globe through their Facebook page. Sitara Krishnakumar and her brand Project Malabaricus had to cancel a series of their concert for U.S. and South East Asia. Being home they composed Song of Valour, a tribute to the health workers. "The music video was stitched together from mobile videos of their respective performances. On Friday night the Democratic Youth Federation of India (DYFI) hosted her on their official page for a live session. The 81,000 listener comments under the live video is a testament to the effectiveness of the medium."[11] On the international jazz day this year the National Centre for the Performing Arts (NCPA), Mumbai, bought together 75 global artistes for the digital performances over three days on Facebook and Instagram pages. Aditi Ramesh, a jazz fusion artist feels, "such gigs are fun as we normally have a limited audience, but during live stream the reach is huge."[12]

Two months (and possibly counting) lockdown has pushed the events like Art Basel Hongkong and Art Dubai to cancel their events and replace them by online viewing rooms. Roshni Vadehra of Vadehra Art Gallery in Delhi, Nupur Dalmia of Gallery Art in Vadodara, Latitude 28 and Kiran Nadar museum of Art, New Delhi; won't be able to launch their shows and will have to wait – no one knows for how long. Commercial galleries have responded speedily to the situation and collaborated to launch a group exhibitions online. 'In Touch' an online exhibition from 10 galleries from India and Dubai started on April 24 and consists of, "12 works from each gallery, the project brings together painters, photographers and sculptors."[13] J Paul Getty museum (U.S.) along with numerous other galleries all over the world have gone online. From Nagpur to New York, illustrators, cartoonist, painters, and graffitists are depicting their current world view through their art and are seeking new ways (web series, Instagram, live stream, Facebook) with the support of art galleries for showcasing their work. The Sunaparanta Centre of Arts in Goa launched a Surviving SQ (self-quarantine) program as an open call to the artist for, "streaming a Share Your Quiet series by New Delhi based video artist Pallavi Paul every Monday on their Instagram handle."[14] Traditionally oriented businesses that depend on walk-ins are in for a bigger challenge, with emerging artists staring at an uncertain future, the dynamics of the industry is gradually changing and upskilling themselves to gear up for the future ahead.

We are the largest film making nation in the world and the madness, expectations, glitz, drama, and vibrancy around a film is unexplainable. Pandemic significantly will impact our film viewing behavior and other economic decisions around it. The collective, social experience of watching films on the big screen in future may have to be redefined. People might stay away from the theatres to avoid large gatherings. This certainly calls for a shift towards viewing films on online platforms. Netflix, Amazon Prime, Hot star, Jio cinema, ZEE 5 and the likes have witnessed a record surge in subscription during the lockdown as these platforms offer a plethora of entertainment options for people locked inside their home to safety. The big movies like Baaghi3 and Angrezi Medium were running in the theatres when lockdown happened, with the shutdown these and many more films waiting for release are going in for huge losses. With theatres remaining close Amazon Prime Video sent ripples through India's entertainment industry by announcing the premiere of Shoojit Sarkar's Gulabo Sitabo, on its platform on June 12 and six other Indian films (Shakuntala Devi biopic) and five regional language films for its 'direct to digital' schedule in the next three months across 200 and more countries. Netflix announced to premier Anurag Kashyap's, 'Choked: Paisa Bolta Hain' on June 5. Even ZEE 5 is premiering Nawazuddin Siddiqui-Anurag Kashyap starrer, 'Ghoomketu,' on May 22. The film is slated for an Eid release on Friday, almost mirroring a theatrical trend. As the chorus around OTT premier grew, the Multiplex Association of India (MAI) urged film makers to release their films in theater and, "respect the exclusive theatrical window, which has been a time tested industry practice,"[15] but the fact is OTT sector in India is steadily growing market and is one segment in the entertainment industry which has done significantly well in the current situation and as Sircar called it, "the dawn of a new era for Indian entertainment."[16]

Sooner or later this pandemic will leave us. But it has surely altered our lives in a way nothing else has in recent history. It has deeply impacted human behavior and concepts. Are we as individuals and as a nation ready for these fundamental changes to cope with the post pandemic world? How best to fit in a world which is and should be changed in many ways post COVID-19? Families, societies, organizations, service providers and even Governments will try and insist that the people follow basic safety protocols in everything they do. And all of this will happen, this is how individuals, companies and government are thinking right now. This then is the New Normal. By early next year if there is no vaccine (or even if there is) we will all know how to be safe and how to carry on with life and work in a brave new world.

References

1. Atwood, Margaret, The Year of Flood.
2. Ratnam, Dhamini; Kaul, Rhythma: 'Social distancing here to stay, small groups may be key;' Hindustan Times, Lucknow, May 04, 2020, p. 6.
3. Ibid.
4. Chakravarty, Parveen; 'Learning to live with Coronavirus,' Hindustan Times, Lucknow, April 27, 2020, p. 8.

5. Ibid.
6. Sukumar, R., 'What You Need to Know Today; Hindustan Times; Lucknow, May 10, 2020, p. 04.
7. Chaturvedi, Hemendra; 'Road to revival seems a tough one,' Hindustan Times; Lucknow May 21, 2020, p. 02.
8. https://www.en.m.wikipedia.org, May 21, 2020, 12:39.
9. Hindustantimes.com, e-paper, May 21, 2020; 15:45.
10. https://www.everythingeperiential.businessworld.in, May 21, 2020; 17:45.
11. http://www.thehindu.com, 'musician go live during covid-19 lockdown,' e-paper, May 22, 2020, 10:00.
12. Kalra, Sanchita; 'International Jazz Day 2020: Observing on the virtual scale,' Hindustan Times, Lucknow, April 30, 2020, p. 12.
13. http://www.livemint.com; May 22, 2020; 15:40.
14. http://www.architecturaldigest.in; May, 22, 2020; 12:45.
15. http://www.hindustantimes.com, 'Release films in theatre……", 23 May 2020, 12:43.
16. http://www.yourstory.com, 'OTTs win over multiplexes….,' 23 May, 2020; 12:56.

9

Innovation as the New Ideator of Post Coronavirus World

— *Dr. Mani Bansal & Dr. A. K. Agarwal*

At the onset of the third decade of the 21st century, COVID-19, spread over 200 countries and territories,[1] has upended the way of life worldwide and has brought many troubles. At present the whole world is counting the days to return to the world that was not inflicted by such ghastly disease. The worldwide political, economic and technical assets have been mobilized to comprehend COVID-19 disease. Impact of this disease shall be long lasting, influencing all domains of human lives. Every individual on the planet needs to be conscious of the measures of our society that will be permanently changed. Life after Coronavirus will be affected by many new twists and turns. Many of these alterations will become instantly the innovative standard, with people familiarizing rapidly to the different ways COVID -19 has impacted their survival. We can look at history as a guide to at least paint a sketch of how the world will evolve after this pandemic settles down. Innovative technologies will be practiced bridging the gap between the physical and virtual worlds.

It is a well-known fact that crises inspire innovation. Similarly COVID-19 disease is an opportunity for innovators not only to protect citizens but also health workers. Digital technology innovations have presented the possibility of improving the ability of human working and the health system response to an epidemic.[2] Latest indication highlights the prospective of establishment of mental health facilities to care for the patients and healthcare providers in dealing with the psychosomatic influence of the COVID-19 disease[3]. Contact tracing apps have been a crucial component of COVID-19 response in many countries.

Innovative India also needs to be a little more compassionate post Corona, and strongly needs to address the problems of the poor. We must harness the talent of the scientists to add value to the local, indigenous ability. During this lockdown and after that, poverty amidst plenty is the tragic experience of the world. It should be the ultimate mission of a nation to achieve economic development for growth and survival. In spite of the great heritage and record of struggles, why did India fall behind in the last centuries? The main causes may be irrational subjective thinking, superficial ritualism, colonial domination and wrong imitation. Gradually we began losing the leadership position. Now this pandemic period is the opportunity when we must regain this position with determined action. We have now an opportunity to start the resurgence of an innovative India. And for this, we need to build new setups to support innovation so that the capital 'I' in India represents Innovation.[3] There is a strong requisite to promote an 'Indian Innovation Movement' now, as we had launched the 'Freedom Movement' to liberate us from British shackles. It will lead India to its rightful place on the world platform.

The landscape of technology and innovation in other services in India is not static. It is continuously evolving. On the human resource front, India has the largest pool of qualified professionals all over the world. Due to this pandemic lockdown, a large cadre of expatriate scientists, technologists and entrepreneurs are rapidly coming back to their home country. As the media reports say, almost the whole world is annoyed with China. And this is what we should en-cash. Some countries are taking back their companies and industries from China and looking for other countries for their establishment. New Innovative India needs to mainly concentrate on youth, which signifies the national power, energy and strength. If youth is properly moulded, they can become the champion of our culture, custodian of our national pride and a trustee of the freedom of the country. Our youth must imbibe the spirit of a true innovator, especially the youth who are airlifted from many countries back home, during this lockdown. After the migration of Indian brains, the government must work out the route from *Saraswati* to *Laxmi*.[4] We must see an expression of entrepreneurship in every citizen of India. How can we induce creative thinking amongst our youth? The young promising inventors can learn a lot from the legendary profession of an inventor like 'Thomas Alva Edison'.

As we know, Edison was granted a record of 1093 patents for inventions ranging from light bulbs, typewriter and electric pen to his phonograph and motion- picture camera. His work methods reveal that the actual key to unlock creativity is an open-minded attitude to learn and determination. Edison always learned from his failures and would enthusiastically record what he had learnt. The lessons that we learn from Edison's life are simple. Challenge the assumptions continuously. Do not have a preset or prejudiced mind. Let the windows of your mind be always open. Second, patience and perseverance pays. Third, nothing is final. Strive for creating products that are better than the best. And displace your products yourself. Finally, you can learn more from your failures than you can from your succcss. So do not bc afraid to fail and takc risks. Innovators arc those who do not know that it cannot be done. Indian history is full of such innovators. There is a strong need to highlight inspiring stories of such innovators. Such stories demonstrate the point that even in India, people, who have done 'out of the box thinking' have won and achieved immensely. During his ministerial period of Ministry of Personnel, Public Grievances and Pensions, Mr. Arun Shorie had organized an inspirational series of dialogues on "Ideas That Have Worked".[5] In this series, several people spoke. N R Narayan Murthy spoke of how by sum of Rs.10,000 in his small 700 square feet apartment, he began to dream of building Infosys. Its market capitalization, at one point of time, was more than Rs.60,000 crores. Infosys has become a pride of the nation today. We can take some more examples such as Mukesh Ambani's Reliance refinery at Jamnagar, Dr. Kurien's white revolution, E. Sreedharan 760 km Konkan railway project, Chandrababu Naidu's work; he has converted Hyderabad into Cyberabad within no time and Ratan Tata's automobile industry. The simple message is that we have done in the past and can do it now for India, in all fields, in all sectors.

During the lockdown, the central government announced emergency relief funds to make poor people independent. There is no doubt that it might be beneficial, if authorities work in a transparent manner. To materialize this, we must create a new value system, where problem solving for the poor and disadvantaged becomes a national mission. Such contributors to this national mission must be reckoned as national heroes. How can we change our mindset and value systems? Technologies developed by local artisans, craftsmen, potters, farmers, weavers etc., are considered as traditional. Such technologies are never involved in the fabric of modern technology. Our challenge in India is to be truly 'inclusive' of our population in the National Innovation Movement and not 'exclusive' to the privileged few. At this point we would like to emphasize that the future of India can be built by keeping in mind and practicing three things, which are encapsulated in the world 'TI'. Firstly, 'TI' stands for 'Think India'. We must have India in our hearts and minds. As someone had said, India's response to WTO should be WTI, that is, 'We Think for India'. The second meaning of 'TI' is 'Team India'. We all need to work, breathe and strive forward as a team. 'TI' also stands for 'Total Innovation'. This means making India truly innovative by altering its public, legal and financial structures.[6]

The COVID-19 virus has significantly changed the outlines of professional life. At present to maintain social distancing, home has become the new office and the Internet is the new meeting room. Unlike software engineers and corporate professionals, teachers and many others are also adapting to these changes. Different community people have innovated to continue their work in these unusual times by different ways to contribute to the fight against COVID-19. Film stars are making inspiring videos to spread the appropriate message of staying at home; many singers are holding online concerts; Chess players are playing digital chess games. Thus the workplace is going "digital first".

If we talk about the education sector, most classes, conferences, meetings are now organised via video conferencing on zoom, google meet, skype, etc. to maintain social distancing. In every sector where social distancing is strictly required video conferencing has become a boon. In the education sector it is being used for conducting online internal exams to complete the academic calendar. The Government of India has also started efforts such as the 'DIKSHA Portal' to help teachers and volunteers to boost e-learning and awareness. 'SWAYAM Portal' is aimed to improve education access, equity and quality. 'E-Pathshala', which is accessible in many languages, offers access to numerous e-books and other educational material. Courses on iGOT have been launched for Doctors, Nurses, Paramedics, Hygiene Workers, Technicians, Auxiliary Nursing Midwives (ANMs), State Government Officers, Civil Defence Officers, Various Police Organisations, National Cadet Corps (NCC), Nehru Yuva Kendra Sangathan (NYKS), National Service Scheme, Indian Red Cross Society, Bharat Scouts and Guides and other volunteers at the stage, which have helped to equip our frontline warriors with capabilities to fight the Coronavirus Pandemic by getting just in time knowledge and skill sets to help tide over the present crisis.[7] Thus technological innovations in the educational system are impacting significantly at all levels. Online courses, educational software, social networking tools, and many other emerging technologies are replacing the outdated classroom atmosphere. There is a need to develop strategies and procedures to manage and use technology in education and to assess the impact of such technological innovations on students, teachers, and schools.

Another sector in which innovation is emerging fast is health. The COVID-19 disease has highlighted that India, a country which has limited resources; needs to work on health solutions at low budgets and at a huge scale. It may position India as a guiding light for worldwide efforts to ensure the health and welfare of humanity. Innovators have come forward and are making it possible to improve technologies along with cost cutting measures. They have innovated economical COVID-19 test kits, indigenously built ventilators, prototypes of isolation wards, Personal Protective Equipment (PPE) and many more arsenals that India is using to conquer the battle against the fatal spread of COVID-19 virus. One of the prime equipment-ventilator, a life support system which provides an imitating flow of natural breath to COVID-19 infected patients, when suffering from scarcity, was created by many startups across the country. Nocca Robotics (incubated at IIT-Kanpur), Aerobiosys Innovations (incubated at IIT Hyderabad) and AgVa Healthcare are developing low cost, easy to use, and portable ventilators which need medical regulatory approval from ICMR (Indian Council of Medical Research) before they could be deployed. Similarly, when the scarcity of COVID- 19 test kits arose, Pune based MyLab Discovery Solutions developed low cost and fast diagnostic test kits. They got the clearance for indigenously manufacturing Covid-19 test kits from ICMR and claimed to screen and detect the infection within 2.5 hours, compared to more than seven hours taken by existing protocols.

In the series of healthcare scarcity the lack of PPE has turned out to be another unaffordable crisis. Our frontline warriors like doctors, nurses, hospital workers, sweepers and others from across the world are facing the scarcity of PPE kits. Many organizations and startups across the nation have come forward and contributed in development of low cost solutions. IIT-Roorkee's Tinkering Labs developed a protection shield at manufacturing cost of Rs. 45 per shield, which can be further reduced with large scale production.[8] IIT-Bombay has made a portable UltraViolet Sanitizing device that can disinfect currency notes, gadgets and similar other items. Indian Army's Corps of Electronics and Mechanical Engineers (EME) have invented a remote-controlled trolley for the use of healthcare workers, to deliver essential items to frontline healthcare staff. To make it more helpful, the trolley comes equipped with a washbasin and dustbin.

The most pertinent thing to research about at present is the invention of the vaccine of COVID -19. Many countries are delving very deep into their research pool but nothing substantial has come out. Countries are looking for innovating with people, process, technologies etc. Innovation can also take the form of flipping a disadvantage into an advantage. Not being a rich country has its advantages for business. Some Indian companies are seeing their business model in it. It is a hard time for the whole world. One such insight is the need to learn from multiple and diverse sources. This is necessary because the situation and problems we confront today demand composite responses and solutions. We might want to study history and biology. As we study more, we will be able to grasp the underlying structures of diverse disciplines and use that insight to enhance the quality of our learning. Analogy has great relevance in our life and work, as we will certainly discover. We believe that this varied exposure provides the mind with stimuli that triggers 'out of the box' or creative thinking. Making connections with seemingly unrelated subjects is a powerful tool, especially in today's world that makes demands on people to be innovative.

To promote innovation in India, the Central government has launched several campaigns on its portal http://innovate.mygov.in.[9] It describes that "Innovate India" is an exclusive platform to display, promote and identify innovations happening across the nation. It has been launched in collaboration with AIM-NITI Aayog and MyGov. All Indian citizens are eligible to share their innovative ideas on this platform. All submitted ideas will be evaluated for adoption and those selected will be suitably rewarded. There are hundreds of innovations that have caught the attention of the Central government and each proposal is being looked into carefully.

Indian government along with the state governments is boosting up efforts to combat the disaster in every way possible. The country is already under lockdown and emergency helplines have been initiated, central and state governments have also developed several mobile applications to make citizens conscious of the current scenario and to track the spread of novel coronavirus. The Indian government has officially launched its COVID-19 tracking app, *Aarogya Setu* (means "bridge to health" in Sanskrit), for both Android and iOS users. The app has been developed by the National Informatics Centre and available in 11 Indian languages.[10] The objective of the app is "augmenting" efforts to "proactively" inform the citizens about the "best practices and relevant advisories pertaining to the containment of COVID-19". It has been made mandatory for citizens living in containment zones, government and private sector employees to download this app. By using a phone's Bluetooth and location data, this app lets users know if they have been near a person with Covid-19 by scanning a database of known cases of infection. The data is then shared with the government. "If you've met someone in the last two weeks who has been tested positive, the app analyses your risk of infection based on how recent it was and its vicinity, and recommends actions". This app does collect this information, as well as your gender, travel history and whether you're a smoker, without making your name and number public. Food delivery start-ups such as Zomato and Swiggy have also made it mandatory for all staff.

The occurrence of the COVID-19 disease has globally created countless challenges to the economy and people's daily lives and will have far-reaching consequences beyond the spread of the disease. At the same time, this crisis has strongly derived creativity and innovation; which are already being observed at each level within the country, whether it is institutional, organizational, and individual. Thus, the pandemic has been a trigger for the innovative minds to create better means to deal with the unprecedented situation by putting their knowledge of technology to optimum use. Innovation has been the survival and evolution plank for the humankind since beginning and even in this time of crisis, it may help us to sail through and devise ways to adapt to the New Normal.

References

1. World Health Organization; "Coronavirus disease 2019 (COVID-19): Situation report-78. Geneva: WHO"; 2020.
2. Reeves JJ, Hollandsworth HM, Torriani FJ, Taplitz R, Abeles S, Tai-Seale M, et al.; "Rapid response to COVID-19: Health informatics support for outbreak management in an academic health system". J Am Med Inform Assoc 2020. pii: ocaa037.
3. Zhou X, Snoswell CL, Harding LE, Bambling M, Edirippulige S, Bai X, et al. The role of telehealth in reducing the mental health burden from COVID- 19. Telemed e Health 2020; 26: 377-9.
4. Mashelker R. A., "Innovation as a way of life", University News Vol. 43, July 11-17, 2005, page 15-17.
5. Sharma S. K. &Sharma U. (2015), Discovery of North East India, Mittal Publication, ISBN 81-8324-034-8.
6. Government of India launches a training module for management of COVID- 19 named 'Integrated Government Online training' (iGOT) portal on DIKSHA platform of MHRD, 09 April; 2020. Accessed from: https://pib.gov.in/PressReleaseIframePage.aspx?PRID=1612437.

7. Bhatia S. & Alexander S, 'Covid-19 shows why we need a healthcare reboot for India', 30 Mar 2020, Accessed from: https://www.livemint.com/politics/policy/will-covid-19-prompt-health- reboot-11585497828527.html.
8. Basu S. D., IIT Roorkee develops low-cost face shields to be used by AIIMS Rishikesh for tackling COVID-19, Apr 03, 2020, Accessed from: https://economictimes.indiatimes.com/news/politics-and-nation/iit-roorkee-develops-low-cost-face-shields-to-be-used-by-aiims-rishikesh-for-tackling-covid-19/articleshow/74971993.cms?from=mdr
9. Launched by Government of India to encourage entrepreneurs to come up with innovative solutions for new India, Accessed from: https://innovate.mygov.in/.
10. Ananth V., "Government requests social media platforms to promote Aarogya" Setu. 2020. Accessed from: https://economictimes.indiatimes.com/tech/software/governmentrequests-social-media-platforms-to-promote-aarogya-setu/ articleshow/75080073.cms, accessed on April 12, 2020.

10

The Changing 'Face' of Fashion in A Post Pandemic Era

— *Dr. Anantdeep Grewal*

Abstract

The COVID -19 pandemic has altered the social and economic structure of the world. The world is going through a medical as well as an economic crisis. We are witnessing a unique historical event, the outcome of which is still not clear except for the fact that the world will not remain the same as we emerge from it. Fashion is related to both society and the economy, hence it is but inevitable for fashion to go through major structural changes post COVID -19. While we will have to make some functional changes in our dressing up due to new social norms, the fashion industry too will adapt itself with the economic depression that is anticipated to follow the pandemic. In view of this it becomes necessary to study the effects of COVID 19 on contemporary fashion world. Although it is not possible to accurately predict the course that fashion will take post this pandemic, some assumptions can be logically made when compared to past events of similar nature and social changes that we are witnessing at present times. In this paper I would be exploring some possible changes in fashion practices as well as in the fashion industry that might be visible in the near future. Predictions made in this paper will be based on some valid examples from history and current developments that are seen around the globe.

Introduction

There is no denying that COVID-19, along with other industries, has also hit the fashion industry quite hard. Sales and production of at least two seasons have been majorly affected by the ongoing pandemic. Experts around the world are desperately looking for measures to minimise the losses and designers must be working on new collection that somehow suits the fresh demand.[1] The call of the time insists one to ponder on the new requirements of the fashion industry post the pandemic. 'Fashion' is the style in clothing, hairstyle, accessories etc. which is popular at a particular time.[2] Throughout history, people have followed fashion traits which reflected their society and which were mostly based on their customs, religion, geographical area, climatic conditions and available technology along with social, economic and political factors of that period. Fashion is ever changing. Major events in history always change the fashion of the times. If we study the developments in fashion during the two World Wars, we would find that hemlines of skirts raised and flouncy skirts became more popular due to rationing of material and as women in the western countries came out to work for the first time in great numbers, some of them started wearing trousers as they were more comfortable for working than the traditional dresses.[3]

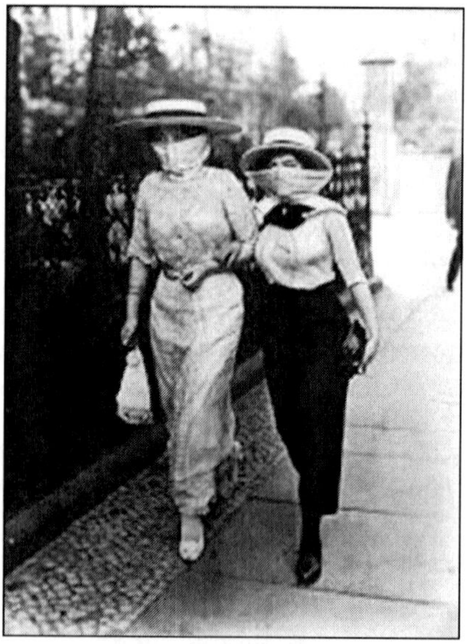

Fashionable women during 1918 to 1920

Global experts of different fields agree that COVID-19 is a major turning point in history but still predictions at present are based on mere speculation as the world has never seen anything of this magnitude. There have been pandemics before but unlike COVID-19 nothing had managed to bring the world to an unprecedented halt resulting in global economic recession which is compared to the 'Great Depression' of the 1930's.[4] If we look at the changes in the outfits brought by one of the recent pandemics, the infamous 'Spanish Flu', we can to some extent judge how society is going to react post COVID-19. The Spanish Flu pandemic started around January 1918 and lasted till about December 1920. It is believed that over 500 million people were infected and around 50 million died.[5] Similar to present practices, social distancing during Spanish Flu was practiced and people also wore masks while stepping out of their homes. Fashionable women sometimes hid their (ugly) masks under a lace veil and made it their fashion statement. Production of masks was done at a large scale and people wore masks even at their workplaces. These are some of the social adaptations that we are witnessing during COVID-19 pandemic too. Masks during early twentieth century were basic in structure and were mainly worn for medical purposes, especially surgery, by doctors to avoid the open wound getting infected by airborne bacteria. In 1910, after the outbreak of pneumonic plague

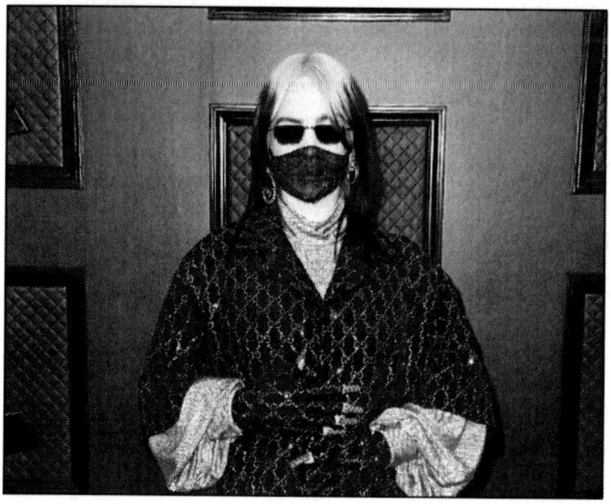

Billie Eilish in mask and gloves at Grammys 2020

in North-east China, the authorities advised the people to wear gauze-and-cotton masks.[6] Later on western countries too adopted it during the outbreak of Spanish Flu. However, the mask in the East Asian countries emerged as a symbol of social responsibility over the years while it was abandoned by the western society. Not until recently masks made a reappearance in the wake of health concerns over air pollution. Brands like Off- White, Palm Angels, Bathing Ape and Fendi have included masks in their accessories and brands like Nemen x Airinum provide breathing masks to counter air pollution.[7] However, these masks are not equipped to protect one from micro-organisms like viruses. Demand for N 95 masks is on the rise as it is considered much safer in the present times.

Since it will be a while for the global population to be vaccinated, we are inclined to infer that social distancing will become part of modern society. Such structural changes have already started in modern society like masks and gloves becoming an essential accessory. However, unlike during the Spanish Flu pandemic, face mask in the future will become more common, safer and yet fashionable. Designer, Masha Ma from China, enhanced the look of the mask by embellishing it with Swarovski crystals for her Paris show in 2015, while Gucci accessorised Billie Eilish for the Grammys 2020, with a mask and gloves to match, to put across the message that "her body is her own, for her eyes only."[8] Both these examples are of masks being used as a style statement and not as any protective gear. With the outbreak of COVID-19 this attitude towards masks will soon change and it will become a lifeline of fashionistas around the globe. Not only designers but regular brands too have started supplying masks to their customers.

In fact, fake designer masks in China are already making an appearance in the market, indicating the growing demand for fashionable masks. Another accessory that will make a comeback is - hand gloves. It should not be surprising to see breezy cotton gloves soon sharing display cabinets with their warmer counterparts, the snow gloves. Although gloves have been around since prehistoric times and already considered a fashion accessory in the colder countries. In the present scenario demand for breezy gloves from the hotter regions of the world too can be anticipated. Clear eyeglasses could be an additional necessity for our future Diva's and Dandies. Like gloves, goggles have been around for centuries now but the need for fashionable safety goggles may also rise, especially for indoor air- conditioned gatherings. With all these additional nitty-gritties, both men and women will be requiring spacious bags. Satchel bags will be more than just a fashion statement of the coxcombs. Although bags are not new to the fashion world for both sexes but it may become a necessity for men as well. As most of face would be covered with masks and the only part visible would be the eyes, eye-makeup may uplift the cosmetic industry. Otherwise there would be less demand for cosmetics as people would not be stepping out of their homes for either work or pleasure.

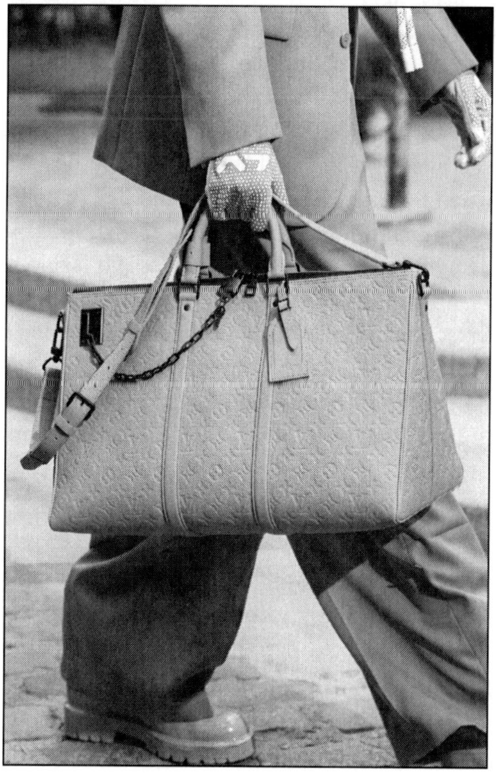

Fashionable bags for men

Besides the Spanish Flu, the COVID-19 outbreak may also have an economic impact similar to The Great Depression of the 1930's, which indicates that people in general will be left with very little spending power.[9] This will impact fashion directly, at least in case of the masses. The pinch of the downward spiral effect of demand and sales ratio is already felt by brands across the world.[10] People would like to spend on essentials, leading to preference towards functional outfits with neutral colours. In similar scenarios neutral colours and classic cuts are usually more in demand as such garments do not stand out and can be repeated multiple times and have style longevity.[11] Classic cuts never go out of fashion and do not look outdated in any setting. Neutral colours can be worn at any time of the day and provide flexibility in usage. Moreover, if garments are cut in classic styles they tend to last longer and are made with less wastage, and neutral colours are dyed cheaper than non-conventional colours. However, fashion is the domain of the rich and it would be one of the last expenses that they will compromise on. The rich demand protection with styles, hence luxurious protection in the form of germfree travel, stylish masks and risk-free holiday options are desired by them.[12] Likewise, when they stay home, they would like to do it in style too. As the ongoing pandemic has cancelled or postponed many socialising, travelling and business plans of the fashionable class, it would not be unreasonable to think that they would desire to lavishly dress up even at home. Under such condition there would be a segment of consumer who would demand overly stylish garments, especially to beat the COVID-19 blues. Garments with brighter colours and elaborate embellishments may also be seen in the coming trends.

Homes, for most, are their comfort zones and in the present state, the overwhelming number of people around the world are confined to their houses, so it is but natural to give preference to comfort over glamour. If we go by the trends on Twitter and Instagram, we may find clues to upcoming trends of comfort wear. Lounge wear with comfortable footwear seems to be the mantra of future fashion. People are not only joking about dreading to wear their uncomfortable jeans and heels and posting pictures on social media showcasing their comfortable sweatpants, but the sales figure of the last two months also points towards this growing trend.[13] Sales of sweatpants with elasticated waistbands has increased and demand for sneakers as compared to other footwear is also on the rise. Lately a feministic trend towards discarding high heels, especially in formal settings like award functions, was becoming a movement.[14] With this worldwide lockdown and an increasing number of people working from home the trend has been accelerated and comfortable footwear along with comfort wear is in demand. The recent trends of dressing of the youth is another indication towards this growing preference.

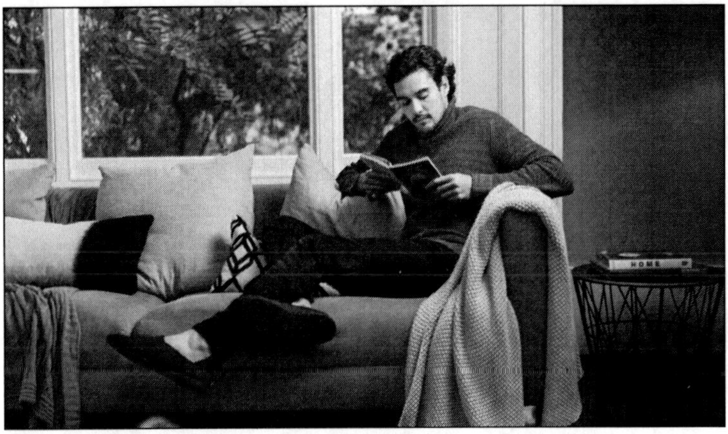

Comfortable lounge wear and shoes are in demand

The mode of socialising is fast changing into Zoom meetings and WhatsApp video callings. Virtual reality is another area that is now explored by people much more than before.[15] The social media interaction gives us an immense control over the perception of our social image. Various filters can create desirable changes in one's features and body shapes without sweating it out or burning a hole in their pockets. With these perfect avatars of themselves there will be truly little motivation to upgrade their wardrobe, or at least not bother with what is not seen through the frame of the camera. Therefore, it would not be too bold to imagine that hairstyles, headgears and trendy tops would be more in demand than the lower garments. Hairstyles, eye makeup and headgear in the coming times have a potential to lead the fashion trends more than the garments themselves. Chances of individual style statements to grow in the coming years also has potential, especially as social media influencers will lose their grip due to lack of impressive content. There would be no events to attend and travelling destinations to explore so social media influencers will struggle to upload content at the same rate that they were initially doing. This may lead to self-exploration and rise in individual fashion statements on part of the young followers.

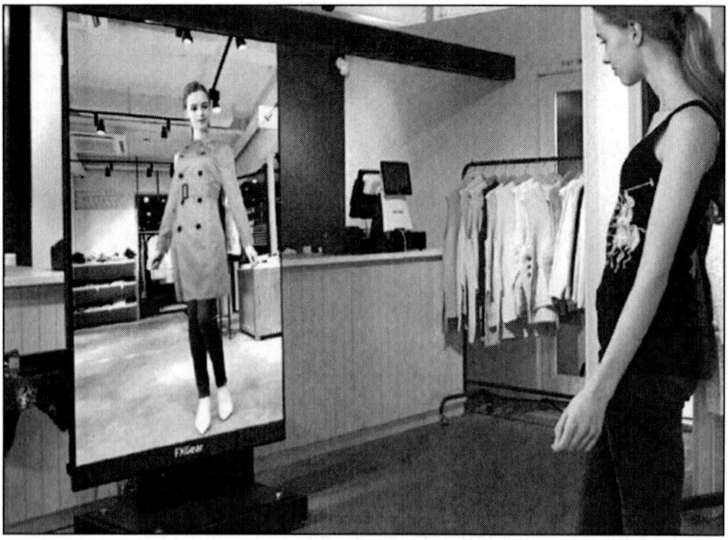

Virtual fitting room

Designer brands are cancelling fashion shows and other events related to them, which were like a ritual with them for many decades now.[16] Fashion weeks too are facing similar adversities as buyers and fashion writers are unable to travel and attend them. As there has been almost negligible sales in the months of March, April and May 2020, leading design houses are rethinking their production and marketing strategies. Lockdowns have highlighted the environmental harm that human intervention has been doing since ages. Designer brands like Gucci are also keeping in mind environmental damage control as they have realised that it is the production part of the garments that harms the environment most. They have decided to hold limited fashion shows in the future, hence bringing out lesser designs per year.[17] Fast fashion,[18] which is a trend of the new millennium is one of the major contributors towards environmental pollution from the fashion world.[19] With COVID-19 this trend neither seems economically viable now nor environmentally sustainable. However, to cut costs the fashion industry may take the help of technology. Automation in the fashion industry will become the norm in the manufacturing units and shopping online will be the preferred choice of the consumer. In fact, brands like Marks & Spencer and Van Heusen have already started providing home delivery services in countries like India too. There will be two parameters on which conscious consumers will base their choices; the health conscious will fear the contamination of the product during its manufacturing and morally conscious would not want to risk the health of the manufacturing workers by them being crowded in the compact factories of the developing world. In both these cases, handmade products will take

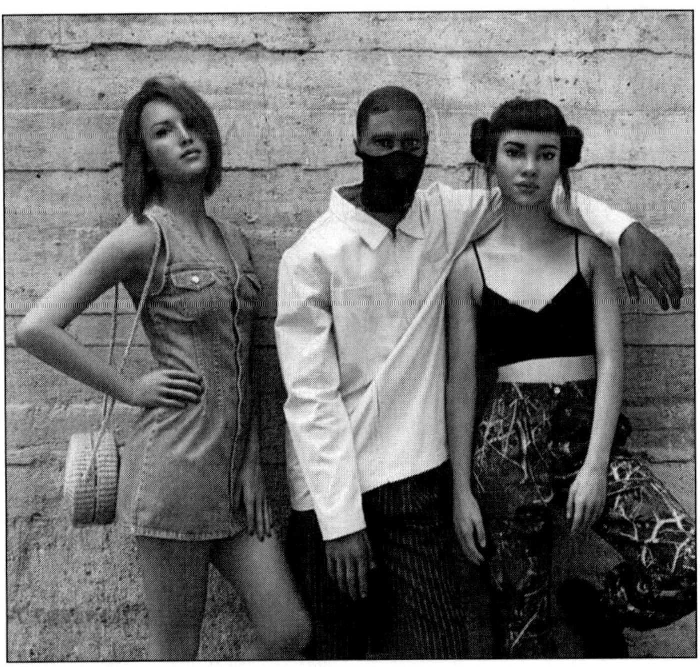

Virtual models in an advertisement

a setback and machine made will prosper. As automation will be used for manufacturing, production will go local. However, this development will negatively affect garment industries in the developing nations. Online shopping may hit the retail outlet hard as brands might provide services of 'Virtual Fitting Rooms' or similar software.[20] Chances of fashion shows and models going virtual are quite high as fashion world has already started moving in that direction.[21] Antimicrobial fabric[22] may also pick up demand as future consumers would like to dress up in safer fabrics. We might see fashionistas bidding farewell to fast fashion, the wasteful and environmentally harmful trend of the twenty-first century. However, it should not be assumed that the Instagram generation will give up so easily on their social media fashionista imaging. In fact, a new life will be given to the custom-made designer wear as CAD/CAM and 3D printers will eventually make single piece manufacturing cost effective. Overall technology is where, like other industries, fashion too will turn to for survival and relevance.

The new changes that are foreseen in the fashion world will be based on four main factors- Health, Environment, Economy and Technology. The future consumers would prefer to wear safe and environment friendly garments and accessories which are easy on their pockets. Technological innovation is what will make this possible. Intervention of new age technology will be seen in every sphere of fashion like advertising, manufacturing and sales. Emphasis will be more on accessories than garments as they will become more a necessity rather than fashion. However, to some extent all these changes will drain glamour out of fashion. In the past few years high end fashion was almost within reach of the common people but with these new developments will again take it into a different realm becoming a niche for the rich.

References

1. Holland, Oscar, 'Gucci abandons 'worn-out ritual' of fashion seasons as the industry looks inward', *CNN*, Updated 26th May 2020, https://edition.cnn.com/style/article/gucci-fashion-calendar/
2. *Collins English Dictionary*, International Edition, HarperCollins Publishers, 2005, pp. 212-213.

3. Haye, Amy de la and Tucker, Andrew, *COSTUME AND FASHION A CONCISE HISTORY*, 4th edition, Thames & Hudson, 2002, pp. 252-254.
4. Cohan, Peter, 'How COVID-19 Crunch Compares To Spanish Flu, Great Depression', *Forbes*, 6th April, 2020, https://www.forbes.com/sites/petercohan/2020/04/06/how-covid-19-crunch-compares-to -spanish-flu-great-depression/#1505e9a61798
5. *THE SPANISH FLU A HISTORY FROM BEGINNING TO END*, HOURLY HISTORY, 2020, p. 20.
6. Lee, Kam Hing, Wong, Danny Tze-ken, Ho, Tak Ming, and Hoong, Ng Kwan, 'Dr Wu Lien-teh: modernising post-1911 China's public health service', *PMC*, US National Library of Medicine National Institute of Health, Feb 2014, https://www.ncbi.nlm.nih.gov/pmc/articles/PMC4291938/
7. Friedman, Vanessa, 'The Mask', *The New York Times*, 17th March, 2020, https://www.nytimes.com/2020/03/17/style/face-mask-coronavirus.html
8. Friedman, Vanessa, 'The Mask', *The New York Times*, 17th March, 2020, https://www.nytimes.com/2020/03/17/style/face-mask-coronavirus.html
9. Cohan, Peter, 'How COVID-19 Crunch Compares To Spanish Flu, Great Depression', *Forbes*, 6th April, 2020, https://www.forbes.com/sites/petercohan/2020/04/06/how-covid-19-crunch-compares-to -spanish-flu-great-depression/#1505e9a61798
10. AU -Testa, Jessica, AU -Friedman, Vanessa and Paton, Elizabeth· 'The Fashion World, Upended by Coronavirus', *The New York Times*, published on March 4, 2020 Updated March 9, 2020, https://www.nytimes.com/2020/03/05/style/the-rich-are-preparing-for-coronavirus-differently.html?action=click&module=RelatedLinks&pgtype=Article
11. AU - Cooper, Tim, AU - Hill, Helen, AU - Kinmouth, J, AU - Townsend, Katherine, AU - Hughes, M, *Design for Longevity: Guidance on Increasing the Active Life of Clothing* , Jan 2013, p-15, https://www.researchgate.net/publication/313479112_Design_for_Longevity_Guidance_on_Increasing_the_Active_Life_of_Clothing
12. Williams, Alex and Bromwich, Jonah Engel, 'The Rich Are Preparing for Coronavirus Differently', *The New York Times*, Published on March 5, 2020 Updated March 9, 2020, https://www.nytimes.com/2020/03/05/style/the-rich-are-preparing-for-coronavirus-differently.html?action=click&module=RelatedLinks&pgtype=Article
13. Gorman, Alyx, 'After months of elasticated waistbands, will we ever give up comfortable clothes?', *The Guardian*, International Edition, 18 May 2020, https://www.theguardian.com/fashion/2020/may/19/after-months-of-elasticated-waistbands-will-we-ever-give-up-comfortable-clothes.
14. Crocker, Lizzie, 'How High Heels Became a Feminist Issue at Cannes', *Daily Beast*, published on 19th May 2015, updated on 14th Apr, 2017, https://www.thedailybeast.com/how-high-heels-became-a-feminist-issue-at-cannes.

15. Biswas, Atanu, 'In the world of virtual reality', *The Statesman*, 30th May, 2020, https://www.thestatesman.com/opinion/in-the-world-of-virtual-reality-1502894312.html

16. Hitti, Natashah, 'Gucci abandons "worn-out ritual" of seasonal fashion shows', *de zeen*, 29th May 2020, https://www.dezeen.com/2020/05/29/gucci-seasonless-fashion-news/

17. Roberts-Islam, Brooke, 'Alessandro Michele's Gucci Announcement: A Leap Towards Sustainability Or A First Step?', *Forbes*, 30th May, 2020, https://www.forbes.com/sites/brookerobertsislam/2020/05/30/alessandro-micheles-gucci-announcement-a-leap-towards-sustainability-or-a-first-step/#6c93eb2a7317

18. "Fast Fashion is the term used to describe clothing designs that move quickly from the catwalk to stores to meet new trends. The collections are often based on designs presented at *Fashion* Week events. *Fast fashion* allows mainstream consumers to purchase trendy clothing at an affordable price." https://www.investopedia.com/terms/f/fast-fashion.asp

19. Schlossberg, Tatiana, 'How Fast Fashion Is Destroying the Planet', *The New York Times*, 3rd Sept, 2019, https://www.nytimes.com/2019/09/03/books/review/how-fast-fashion-is-destroying-the-planet.html

20. http://zugara.com/virtual-dressing-room-technology

21. Sudevan, Praveen, 'Pixel-perfect models: Virtual influencers could be the future of fashion advertising', *The Hindu*, 9th July, 2019, https://www.thehindu.com/sci-tech/technology/internet/pixel-perfect-models-virtual-influencers-could-be-the-future-of-fashion-advertising/article28331935.ece

22. Veneziale, Erin, 'CAN ANTIMICROBIAL FABRIC STOP THE SPREAD OF VIRUSES?', *Mood Sewciety*, https://www.moodfabrics.com/blog/can-antimicrobial-fabric-stop-the-spread-of-viruses/

11

Brighter Facets of COVID-19: Lessons Learnt by Mankind

— Owais Ismaeil

Abstract

The sudden shock that humanity received at the outbreak of Covid-19 was numbing. Never before had the human race come to such a halt, where all the activities were suspended, everybody was locked down in their homes, across the world a pal of gloom and fear descended as the virus swept across nation after nation. However, seeking a way out in the face of grim situations is a human specialty. The amazing ability to perceive something good even in the darkest of times has kept the human race alive. Since times immemorial, human beings have been rebuilding their lives after devastation. As a community they survive. While the news from all around is about death and dread, this paper seeks to shed light on a few positive sides of the situation, the few glimpses of brighter side effects of lockdown. Realisation, sense of oneness, and a changed attitude for the future are some of them.

Key Words: *Positive, Covid-19, lockdown, brighter, rebuilding.*

Humans have a history of braving challenges since the dawn of civilization. Humanity has wrestled with the greatest challenges like World War I & II and continued to strive against all odds till now.[1] The COVID-19 pandemic is one of the biggest challenges we are facing currently since it does not differentiate between rich and poor, white and black, developed and developing and so on. We are frequently flooded with terrible news of death, anguish, misery, cynical contagion reports, losing jobs and looming economic recession which altogether could lead to depression, anxiety, and fear. However, being on the optimistic side and repeating the history of facing challenges, it has revealed some immense brighter aspects of humanity that we may not have discovered under normal circumstances. Coronaviruses are a huge group of viruses that typically cause mild to moderate upper- respiratory tract illnesses, like the common cold. Three of these viruses, SARS coronavirus (SARS- CoV) that emerged in November 2002, Middle East respiratory syndrome (MERS) that emerged in 2012 and novel coronavirus called SARS-CoV-2 are more serious and fatal.[2] SARS-Cov-2 also called as COVID-19 and declared as global pandemic on March 11, 2020 by World Health Organization (WHO) is shaking whole world.[3] Most of the nations including India is managing to curtail the spread of this deadly virus by imposing lockdown and it has been found the only productive way apart from taking precautionary measures to control the spread of infection.[4] Analysing the reactions in response to the COVID-19 pandemic and taking into consideration the drastic decline in human activities, analysts, doctors and researchers have noticed some curious and surprisingly positive side effects of this abrupt shift in human behaviour. It was observed that sky became clearer and bluer, accident rates decreased drastically[5], crime rate was enormously reduced, some other infectious diseases disappeared from the hospitals. Although people were forced to stay home but to a larger extent it reunited family members and led them to work together, share their experiences and developed some new skill sets.[6] This chapter describes the brighter facets of COVID-19 and the lessons we have learnt to be good humans which we had forgotten somehow due to our material desires. It taught us that sufferings are common to us and we should never ignore the suffering and misery of our fellow human beings and other creations of God.

The Covid Sweep

Novel coronavirus (SARS-Cov-2) also called as COVID-19 was first reported in the month of December 2019, in China's Wuhan district and it was declared as global pandemic on March 11, 2020 by World

Health Organization (WHO).[7] Its infection transmitted very rapidly across the globe affecting millions of people of all age groups. Coronaviruses are a huge group of viruses that typically cause mild to moderate upper-respiratory tract illnesses, like the common cold. The infection is transmitted by inhalation or contact with infected droplets and its incubation period is believed to range from 2 to 14 days. In most of the cases, the symptoms are typically dry cough, tiredness, fever, sore throat, breathlessness and more recently loss of taste is found to be a significant symptom of the disease. It has been found to be mild in most of the people with exceptions of elderly and those who are already with co-morbidities. Its progression has been found to result in pneumonia, acute respiratory distress syndrome (ARDS) and multi organ dysfunction. There are 4 species of corona virus family namely HKU1, NL63, 229E and OC43 that have been found transmitting in humans causing mild respiratory disease.[8] Possible vaccines and some specific drug treatments are under investigation. There are several promising clinical trials underway and we are hopeful for the success. The COVID-19 pandemic is a crucial global health crisis of our time and the greatest global humanitarian challenge the world has faced since World War-II.[9] The virus has spread widely, and the number of cases are surging like wild fire. India acted promptly by implementing a proactive, nationwide lockdown, with the goal of knocking down the curve. According to lockdown announcement in India, all academic institutions, industries, markets and all public places were closed until further notifications and several announcements were made and are still being made relaxing the essentials/services in a phased manner. Being a highly populated country, complete lockdown was the only solution to contain the spread of infection to a larger extent.[10] Along with an unprecedented human toll, COVID-19 has elicited a deep economic, health and social price. Everything was closed all of a sudden and everybody was advised to maintain social distancing, this is something which utmost modern human brains would have never thought, but yes it happened in 2020, where we are not able to fly for months, where we are not allowed to celebrate together our festivals. However, we have lessons to learnt from such pandemics, each one of us need to ask ourselves, how much harm we are doing daily to our environment. With this rapid and drastic decline in human activity in response to the COVID-19 pandemic, analysts, doctors and researchers have noticed some curious and surprisingly positive side effects of this abrupt shift in human behaviour.[11] The crisis brought home many forgotten lessons and reminded us of the values earlier highly cherished but lost in the mad race of materialism. Human beings that were almost turning into machines away from the qualities of heart somehow got their feelings and humanity back when faced with collective death.

"In the midst of chaos, there is also an opportunity."

–Sun Tzu

Positive impact on Environment

The coronavirus lockdown has greatly rejuvenated our environment. Decline in human activity and machines has helped a lot in improving the environmental conditions. Factories were either shut or minimally operating, public transport as well as private vehicle movement was minimized to a significant level, air traffic was mostly shut off, huge gathering and parties were no more allowed during the lockdown. Reports have suggested that reduction in industrial and transport emissions and effluents has greatly improved the quality of air, soil and water. The month of May, which generally records peak carbon emissions due to the decomposition of leaves, has recorded what might be the lowest levels of pollutants in the air since the 2008 financial crisis. Furthermore, there has been a 25% decline in energy use and emissions in China over two weeks which is likely to decrease the overall annual carbon emissions of the country by 1 per cent.[12] In India, the results were comparable, March 22 was declared as the 'Janata Curfew', following which, a significant drop in air pollution levels was recorded across the country. Cities like Delhi, Kolkata Bengaluru, and Lucknow saw their average Air Quality Index (AQI) staying within two digits. Air pollution levels in India, especially in New Delhi has been found to be reduced by 50% due to lockdown. Figure 1 shows that air pollution over northern India particularly in Delhi NCR has been recorded a 20-year-low for this time of the year. The figure indicates the pollution level in Delhi NCR during 2019 and 2020.[13]

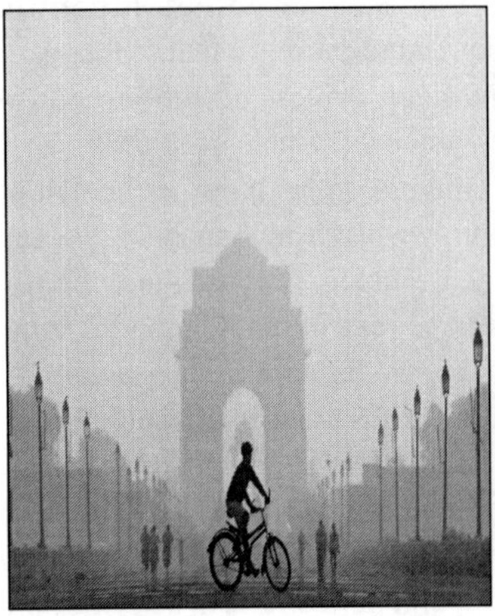

Source: CNN

The India Gate war memorial in New Delhi on 20 October, 2019

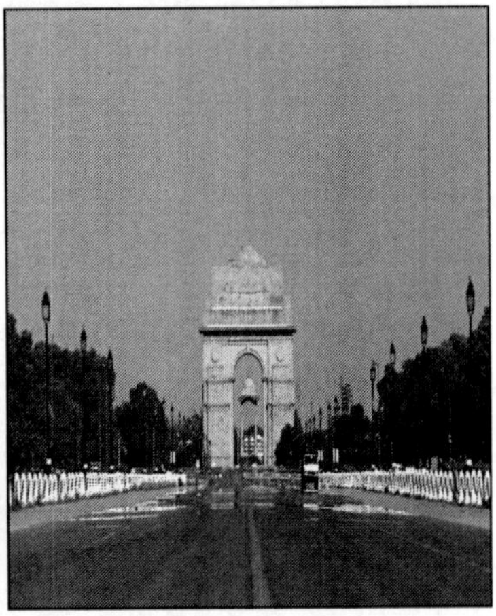

Source: The New York Times

The India Gate war memorial in New Delhi on 02 May, 2020

In addition, the instance of cleaner air was seen; on April 3rd, residents of Jalandhar, Punjab woke up to a view of the Dhauladhar mountain range, a rare feat in normal times, considering the distance between the two places lying almost 213 kilometers apart from each other and in recent memory, it was not visible from the city. Similarly, NCR residents are enjoying a sustained spell of blue skies after more than a decade and are happy to breathe fresh air in their balconies or roof tops.[14]

Since non-essential activities took a break, energy demands have dropped substantially which resulted in improved air quality. Maharashtra, one of the country's most industrialized states, witnessed power demand decline from 23,000 MW to 13,000 MW. Likewise, during this lockdown, petrol sales have plunged by 17 per cent and diesel by 26 per cent.[15]

Water bodies have also been clearing, and rivers such as Yamuna and Ganga have seen significant improvement since a nationwide lockdown was enforced. According to the Central Pollution Control Board's (CPCB) real-time water monitoring data, the average water quality of the Ganga seen in recent days is suitable for bathing, wildlife and fisheries propagation.[16]

It was observed over a period that the pollution control experiments, and rules and regulations were entirely a failure for years. With different tactics of odd and even drives, pollution control vehicles, off-road old vehicles etc., authorities have been trying hard to control the pollution but have failed to do so. Now, lockdown of few weeks compelled us to stay home, work from home, study from home which resulted in minimized outside activities and finally not only controlling pollution to a larger extent but helping in ozone layer healing. In brief, since decades, we humans are degrading all environmental cycles, but COVID-19 has provided a great chance to recycle environmental processes and reenergise the positive waves. Although, our government has made considerable efforts to provide us with clean water and has invested massive amounts of money in filtering and purifying it but, until and unless human activities are minimised and the sustainable environmental measures are adopted, it's very difficult to get the quality from the nature. With the lockdown it looks like the natural reserves which were polluted by humans time to time are now being rejuvenated. In conclusion, the take-home message is that once everyone gets back to normal life, better realization of the environmental, transport and industry regulations should be considered a priority to ease the harmful environmental impacts of human activity.

Proper Sanitization Measures

Our discipline of hygiene has improved enormously. While analysing profoundly, we realized that COVID-19 has come to balance our lives and also fill the gaps in our lifestyle, relationship, universe and nature. Cleanliness is said to be next to divinity. We understand that we keep ourselves hygienic by routine cleansing but from the day we have come to know that to keep this infection away, we have to clean ourselves each time we touch anything or come close to any person or object, we have started following it in letter and spirit. Now, we not only sanitize, disinfect ourselves but we are taking care of things that directly or indirectly belong to us. Without any special occasion or festival, we started to clean our homes and surroundings regularly and to support cleaning up our society and community for a healthy nation.[17] If this realization stays throughout the year, most of the

infections could be contained in the society easily, where you could be the either the source or the protector, choice is yours?

Good Family Relations

When it comes to our family relationships, every one of us must acknowledge that COVID -19 provided us an opportunity to restore and reconnect fully with our family and again we started to restrain our movement to respect our elderly but caring about their health since they are at highest risk. Spending enough time with our family members made us realise that our family is our best supporter no matter whatever the situation is, although it is always there but the sense of feeling is an exceptional experience in this technological era. Parents had more time to enjoy with children, teach them their own experiences, playing board games, experiencing in cooking etc. We realised that there is an opportunity to even work from home. We were listening since long that the time would come when everything will be online and within our reach with the simple click of few buttons on our keyboard. Perhaps COVID-19 is the result of that prediction which our elders already indicated, and we are the witness of this transformation.[18]

In this competitive world, we are always tired because of our busy schedule and COVID-19 seems to have provided us an opportunity to take a deep breath, take some rest and reunify with ourselves to start up afresh. Live a life full of passion and sensations with our loved ones. In short we are not sanitizing and disinfecting ourselves but our thoughts and way of living which is a good start due to bad VIRUS. Although COVID-19 is a deadly virus killing enmass human beings but again the positive part of it is that it is giving us a way of thinking to be hygienic physically and mentally, no virus can damage any of us till we are united and strong and ready to help each other. [19]

COVID-19 Promoted Humanity, Modesty, and Acceptance

COVID-19 has encouraged us to believe and comprehend that we are not the undeniable masters of this world. No matter, if we conquer the highest peaks, dive into the deep seas, slaughter the powerful animals, displace tall trees, the nature can also avenge in her own

ways. It just unleashed an invisible nano creature and we are terrified with panic and anxiety. We are now realising the power of nature, and I believe nations have shun their arrogance of superiority and superpower. Human are now behaving modestly and trying their best possible to save themselves and others from spread of this disease. Its not about disease only. We must be always ready, no matter what the situation is to help each other and behave as humans with great humility. COVID- 19 provided us a glimpse of golden era when we see people coming close to helping one another by fulfilling the needs of others without counting their actions. Now people are easily seen distributing food and other basic items of need without asking for a name or a caste. Even industrialists and celebrities, always busy at making money, have opened their hearts and pockets to help, heal and feed the needy. Everybody is accepted in this pandemic despite of caste, creed, colour. The Governments are making every effort to support and care for its nationals. The leaders and government employees are coming forward to contribute their share of the wages to the needy. All of these are the signs where we can proudly declare that humanity has started breathing again. Government has taken praiseworthy steps by issuing rent relaxation advisory, utility payment plans, EMI Bank deferment and many more. In short, this is an awakening period in which everyone actively does their part to support and assist each other's survival.[20]

Accidents & Crime Rate Reduced

As soon as the COVID-19 started appearing in India, the authorities took an immediate decision of lockdown. They halted public transit, stacked medical gear and ordered more than 1.3 billion residents to stay indoors. The concern was that if COVID-19 spread through densely crowded cities across India, especially its slums, millions would die. The toll could be much worse than in Europe or the United States, where doctors and hospitals are many more per capita. With immediate lockdown and restrictions on movements thousands of lives have been saved nationwide in numerous ways most of us would not have imagined. Since the lockdown was effective, there have been very less road accidents, very few cases of murders and reports of violence against women and fewer suicides.[21]

The Government recorded more than 150,000 road accident deaths in 2018, the latest year for which data are available. By contrast, the U.S., which has higher car ownership per capita, saw more than 36,000 road deaths the same year. Average of about eight people killed on commuter trains per day in the commercial capital Mumbai. As passenger trains stopped on 22 March, eight people have died so far throughout April. Mumbai reported a 20% drop in all non-COVID-19 related deaths last month, compared to March 2019. According to the latest Delhi Police data, the crime rate in the city has dropped considerably. The data between March 15 and March 31 show that most crimes have reduced by half and a few others saw a drop of 80%. Since there are little to no people on the streets because of the lockdown, street crimes and fatal road accidents have fallen, and an increased police presence and closed borders have contributed to a low burglary and vehicle theft rate. Severe checking at the borders has caused a deterrent for criminals from the neighbour states. Robbery, kidnapping and extortion too have plunged tremendously.[22] There is a 44% decrease in crimes compared to last year. There were only 1,890 crimes reported this year compared to last year's 3,416. Cases of molestation of women have reduced from 144 last year to 72 this year. Fighting cases have declined by 65% as most people are confined to their homes. Police presence has increased across the cities and at borders, particularly in hotspots and crime-prone areas. Due to shutdown of shops and other small businesses, drinking alcohol in public has declined to a great extent and the related crimes as well.[23] Although, it is true that we lost many lives due to COVID-19 infection and we had a huge impact on our economy but at the end we are the ones who can build up the economy again, the need of the hour was to revisit our human nature, which we had lost somehow in our busy schedule. Re-energizing ourselves with that modesty and humanity is the brighter facet of COVID-19.

"STAY HOME, STAY SAFE, STAY COOPERATIVE"

References

1. I. Chakraborty, P.Maity, COVID-19 outbreak: Migration, effects on society, global environment and prevention https://doi.org/10.1016/j.scitotenv.2020.138882.

2. Scripps Research Institute. "COVID-19 coronavirus epidemic has a natural origin".
3. Gautam S, Hens L (2020) SARS-CoV-2 pandemic in India: what might we expect? Environ Dev Sustain 22:3867–3869
4. Sneha Gautam (2020), The Influence of COVID-19 on Air Quality in India: A Boon or Inutile, Bulletin of Environmental Contamination and Toxicology (2020) 104:724–726.
5. Bryn Nelson(2020), The positive effects of COVID-19, http://www.bmj.com/
6. Coronavirus lockdown: Crimes in Delhi drop by 80% as people stay indoors, https://www.businesstoday.in/latest/trends/coronavirus-lockdown-crimes-in-delhi-drop-by-80-as-people-stay-indoors/story/400142.html
7. Sneha Gautam (2020), The Influence of COVID-19 on Air Quality in India: A Boon or Inutile, Bulletin of Environmental Contamination and Toxicology (2020) 104: 724–726.
8. National Health Mission Report, Government of Karnataka. https://www.mohfw.gov.in/pdf/FAQ.pdf
9. I. Chakraborty, P.Maity, COVID-19 outbreak: Migration, effects on society, global environment and prevention https://doi.org/10.1016/j.scitotenv.2020.138882
10. Bureau, Our. "PM Modi calls for 'Janata curfew' on March 22 from 7 AM-9 PM". Businessline; 19 March 2020.
11. Bryn Nelson(2020), The positive effects of COVID-19, http://www.bmj.com/
12. Chelsea Gohd, Air pollution over northern India drops amid coronavirus lockdown, https://www.space.com/india-air-pollution-drops-coronavirus-lockdowns.html
13. Chelsea Gohd, Air pollution over northern India drops amid coronavirus lockdown, https://www.space.com/india-air-pollution-drops-coronavirus-lockdowns.html
14. Sarika Panda Bhatt, The Times of India, https://timesofindia.indiatimes.com/blogs/voices/time-to-assess- coronavirus-beyond-cases-and-deaths/
15. Sarika Panda Bhatt, The Times of India, https://timesofindia.indiatimes.com/blogs/voices/time-to-assess- coronavirus-beyond-cases-and-deaths/
16. The Economic Times Report, Lockdown: Health of river Ganga improves https://economictimes.indiatimes.com/news/politics-and-nation/lockdown-health-of-river-ganga-improves/articleshow/74946264.cms
17. Raheel Khan @OFF THE FACE, https://timesofindia.indiatimes.com/readersblog/off-the-face/positive-side-of-COVID-19-11657/
18. Raheel Khan @OFF THE FACE, https://timesofindia.indiatimes.com/readersblog/off-the-face/positive-side-of-COVID-19-11657/

19. Raheel Khan @OFF THE FACE, https://timesofindia.indiatimes.com/readersblog/off-the-face/positive-side-of-COVID-19-11657/
20. Raheel Khan @OFF THE FACE, https://timesofindia.indiatimes.com/readersblog/off-the-face/positive-side-of-COVID-19-11657/
21. Mystery of India's lower death rates seems to defy coronavirus trend, The Economic Times Report, https://economictimes.indiatimes.com/news/politics-and-nation/mystery-of-indias-lower-death-rates-seems-to-defy-coronavirus-trend/articleshow/75346712.cms?from=mdr
22. Report On Business Today, Coronavirus lockdown: Crimes in Delhi drop by 80% as people stay indoors, https://www.businesstoday.in/latest/trends/coronavirus-lockdown-crimes-in-delhi-drop-by-80-as-people-stay-indoors/story/400142.html
23. Report On Business Today, Coronavirus lockdown: Crimes in Delhi drop by 80% as people stay indoors, https://www.businesstoday.in/latest/trends/coronavirus-lockdown-crimes-in-delhi-drop-by-80-as-people-stay-indoors/story/400142.html

12

Covid-19 and Appropriation by the Electronic Media

— *Dr. Archna Rathore*

Covid-19 is certainly the gravest global health crises till date. It was on 11th February 2020 when the WHO proposed this official acronym for the disease caused by the coronavirus. The ongoing researches tell us that COVID-19 is here to stay as we have not been able to invent a vaccine for it, inspite of the first human trial of coronavirus being started on 23rd April 2020. In order to truly understand this disease, it's better to listen from an expert, Dr. Fauchi. He says, "When people ask me what I worry most with regard to emerging infectious diseases, is a respiratory borne illness that easily spreads from person to person, but that has a high degree of morbidity and mortality. And unfortunately, that's the worst nightmare you could have, to have something like that. I mean, there are other diseases; Ebola was frightening, but Ebola gets transmitted only when you are in very close contact with a person who is very, very ill. With this disease, in some respects similar to influenza, it spreads very easily. You can spread it when you are not symptomatic. So it's insidious and treacherous. In that you could spread it easily. The other part about it that's really so different from anything that we've ever faced before, is that if you look at the mortality of seasonal flu, the mortality is about 0.1 percent. That's a lot. And we get used to that morbidity and mortality. But the mortality of this is about ten times that. So, it's a disease that is easily spread, particularly for a certain subset of the population."

He further informs that the things that are the most common, that one really has to latch onto is the sneezing and coughing. If someone is ill, they have got to get themselves out of circulation, because they can spread by droplets, and even by what we call aerosol, which means the drop doesn't go down right away. It hangs around for a bit. So you could come into a room, thinking everything is all right, and then you inhale it. So, this coronavirus disease is something that we cannot take lightly.

The paper stringently sticks to three points when understanding Media's handling of Covid 19 Pandemic.

(1) Theories about the origin of Coronavirus

(2) Theories about how to combat this pandemic

(3) Government policies dealing with this pandemic

In focus here is the stand of the media, whether it works as an agent to give information to the audience or becomes a bigger platform of advertisement of government efforts. Or, it hooks the audience by screening the sleazy and the sensational stuff about coronavirus. It is seen that the channels airing the fake news about the coronavirus do it in such dramatised way that even after declaration by them that this is fake, the visuals do remain with the audience.

Another pertinent point to study is whether the media has lost all the optimism or it's trying to inculcate a ray of hope in the people. It's very interesting to observe how different TV channels or Youtubers choose to air the stories about our current times. In this paper, I have taken the case study of two countries- India and America, vis a vis their Media. We see so many conflicting ideas online, regarding the information about corona virus. And, the horrible by-product of having social media and the internet is, everyone is now an expert, and everyone has an opinion. There's no gainsaying in the dictum, fake news is the one thing that spreads faster than the corona virus. Researchers at Carnegie Mellon University say nearly half the twitter accounts spreading messages about Corona virus are likely to be computerised bots. The study found over 100 false narratives about COVID-19 since January 2020. The goal seems to be generating a division in America.

One of the things that attract different TV channels and YouTube influencers is the 'Conspiracy theories' of where the corona virus actually came from! The first theory that gripped people across the countries was that virus jumped from a bat to human beings. The pandemic could have started as a food thing until it came that those viral videos of people eating bat soups weren't even filmed in China. And then we found out, that virus can't survive cooking anyway. Then there was the theory that the virus was bioengineered in a lab by scientists just to be used as a weapon or a form of population control. This has also not been confirmed as yet. Different channels gave substantial screen time to different theories depending on their whims and fancies.

Pandemic in India and the Media Coverage

If we look at highlights or milestones in the journey of Corona virus in India, starting from 30th January 2020, when India reported the first confirmed case of the Coronavirus infection in the state of Kerala to the 182,143 confirmed cases on 31st May 2020, when this paper is being written, we can come up with these points:

(1) Junta curfew on 22nd March 2020 at the appeal of Prime Minister Mr. Modi and the subsequent lockdowns, starting from 24th March.

(2) Tabligi Jamat emerging as the new Coronavirus hotspot on 31st march 2020.

(3) Prime Minister's address to the nation.

(4) Reverse migration of the labours from their place of work.

(5) Government policies, specially the economic policy and the arrangements for the migrant labours.

Alongwith these points, there's a whole gamut of self- proclaimed and at times, self-made theories about curing the coronavirus disease that keep acquiring screen space in different news channels.

The Janta curfew was lauded by the pro-government TV channels in hyperbolic magnitude while the anti-establishment channels had all the logic to call it a fiasco. The flagrant examples are Republic TV and NDTV India, respectively. It would have been great if the address by the PM could be presented as it was, without the extreme left or right interpretations.

The PM's address on 24th March 2020, announcing the complete 21 day lockdown became the most viewed event in the history of Indian TV, as per the data from TV viewership monitoring agency BARC India. It was aired by all the media houses and gave food for thought to them for many days. The twitter was abuzz with that, the entertainment channels came up with the suitable advertisements and gradually there were short jingles on social distancing and washing of the hands by the celebrities.

Again, the media was divided on the coverage of Tabligi Jamat in India. Some channels took it up as the bait to hold cantankerous debates, mostly one sided. They stuck to inviting some *maulana* representing the Jamat and kept on lambasting him in decibels higher than could be tolerated. While some kept on favouring them and tried hard to give them benefit of doubt, more than could be allowed! There's no doubt that the country needed to know of the whereabouts of Maulana Mohammad Saad but he didn't deserve extended screen hours for days. He became more of a filler. When they had nothing new to air, they succumbed to debating on Saad. Here, the electronic media plummeted to a low.

During this pandemic (COVID-19), we are frequently getting news about the situation of the migrant workers. On one hand, large number of workers have been sent already to their respective places and on the other hand a large population of workers is still waiting for their turn. If we are in a mood to criticise the government or appreciate the efforts made by the government we can choose our news channels/ sources accordingly as both types of information is available in abundance. Some channels are focusing only on the atrocities being inflicted on the bare-feet workers, marching on the unending roads while some are trying to understand the massive administrative acumen involved in managing such whopping population. We, as viewers, need to develop a rationale of our own to perceive things in an impartial manner because this pandemic is not evanescent, it will have its deep down effects.

With media space crowded with so many players, plus the social media and the trending news, it's becoming more and more difficult for the average individual to sift through relevant information. So, they become prisoners of habit and end up watching and following the same set of news channels, newspapers and social media news places. The media houses are able to convey a sense of unity only for very hard facts- like COVID numbers, PM Modi's address to the nation, Economic package information. But beyond that the interpretation is purely biased.

Social media by design is tuned to show content to an individual based on their preferences. So they will slowly and surely keep increasing the tone of news in a particular direction, depending on past viewership, since that's how they grab engagement of users. The most measure metric for social media companies is MAO and DAO-Monthly and daily active users and engagement figures. So they can and are creating a polar world. Their Machine learning algorithms are not and cannot be tested fully and hence are dehumanising the entire environment. What we need is social media to use these Machine learning altos to create a balanced view of the world and navigate people towards that.

We can harness the flexibility and ubiquity of media technologies to increase the public's adherence to the safety measures suggested by global health organizations to combat the spread of COVID-19. In fact, had India (and other countries) created an app to track all visitors to our country from outside, we would have been able to control the spread at source. Now in today's world, it's possible that WHO or similar world bodies focus on tracking app, updates and guidelines. So, for example an Arogya Setu kind of application from WHO, will eliminate all security questions and provide a world view and better data collection, analytics and eventual prescriptive analytics of what next to do.

The question is about the role of media in conveying the information. Whether the information being provided is genuine, positive, and with a common purpose and aim to benefit the people, in general? Or are they indulging in furtherance of their own views, tailored messages? To quote Shri Sandeep Ravivanshi, Divisional Security Commissioner, RPF (Railway Protection Force), "If we talk about the news channels I can say that they don't share a common objective except in making money perhaps. Many are indulged in furthering interest of particular political parties, even at the cost of facts. Some are behaving as mouthpiece of political parties only. Some facts are being exaggerated out of proportion by some channels. Role of Tablighi Jamaat was one of such facts. Some media houses are still propagating unscientific and superstitious practices. Instance of that Saryu cow is one example. Though positive news and stories are surely being shown but negative content far outweighs the latter. The impact is not so positive."

He further goes on to opine that as far as COVID-19 is concerned, most channels have shown good practices to be followed. And they were very effective in that. But there is no agreement on how effective the lockdown has been. Adverse effect of management of COVID-19 on economic development and health system as a whole, finds only passing reference.

Responsible role of media, be it broadcast or social media, could have been to be informative and to create a rational discussion that helps public in opinion making. In other words, media is useful if it helps public to decode government policy, if it helps public to get exposure of outcomes of present socio-political ethos and if it could genuinely connect with the expectations of common people.

Unfortunately the situation is absolutely opposite. Instead of the media making its views and voice as per the aspirations of people, it is the present so called free media that creates groups based on ideology for certain political motives. Interesting aspect of the new face of media is that people have started analysing views of different media and forming their own independent opinion, a more rational one. They receive information and test it, verify it and create logical opinion.

Social media has given a good platform for public debate and spread of ideas and public opinion. Raw multimedia information gives base to genuinely understand the true situation and pressure the government to review their policy. For example, we all are witness to migrant labourers' videos and their sufferings that blatantly defeats government claims and it is forced to review it. If the source is properly verified, then it is a very useful medium. Videos getting viral of hatred and violence aren't from authentic source most of the times; either the video is tampered or edited with mala-fide intention.

Pandemic in America and the Media Coverage

America has an outlandish graph of coronavirus positive cases, from the first confirmed case on 20th January 2020 to 1,788,762 confirmed cases and a ghastly 1,04,356 deaths.

The milestones in USA during this pandemic can be zeroed into these-

(1) Suspension of entry into the USA by anyone who has travelled to China in the past 14 days.

(2) Trump's stimulus package of 2 trillion dollars on 27th March 2020.

(3) Pulling out of WHO funding by Trump, accusing it of mismanaging the pandemic.

(4) Obamagate.

(5) Broad day light murder of George Floyd.

The common sense prevailing amongst the general masses educates them to not rely on any flimsy or casual source. We should give leverage to the information coming out of the health ministry or somebody of the status of a nation head. But now we realise we can't even rely on nation heads also, that too the President of the super power America. To illustrate a few statements by him-

"Corona virus will disappear like a miracle."

"People had nothing to lose by experimenting with hydroxychloroquine."

"Virus can't see you if you don't move."

And his weirdest unlicensed medical opinion- Using ultraviolet rays and injecting disinfectants such as bleach and alcohol.

When confronted by the media and suggested otherwise by his medical team, he covered it all up by saying it was sarcasm! Even the allegedly pro Trump channel, Fox News could not take his side in pontificating such opinions and had to condemn them. Mr. Trump was not far behind denigrating them in his tweet on 18th May 2020, "Fox News is no longer the same. We miss the great Roger Ailes. You have more anti Trump people, by far, than ever before. Looking for a new outlet!"

In an article by Amy Mitchell and Baxter Oliphant, it is stated that most Americans think that media are doing fairly well covering it. "About half of the public (48%) say they've been exposed to at least some made up new information related to the virus." As we can say for our Indian news channels, that they are inclined for or against the political party in power, the same holds true for USA too!

Coming to Obamagate, it is said that the President is reeling politically from his deadly incompetence during the coronavirus pandemic and now he and his sycophants on state TV are trying to distract from that by obsessively spinning wild conspiracy theories about Barrack Obama. When asked even mildly challenging questions in a recent press conference, he walked out of that!

When we talk about media and the COVID-19, the talk shows that were aired on TV as well as YouTube have now gained more substance because people are tired of watching the repeats of the serials. This is when the monologues steal the show and they do come up with something interesting and thought provoking. In this genre, American talk shows dominate the scene, especially the monologues done during this lockdown. Some brilliant examples are 'Late Night with Seth Meyers' that has the big story covered in its segment, 'A Closer Look', 'Jimmy Kimmel's Quarantine Monologue', "The Late Show with Stephen Colbert' and 'The Daily Social Distancing Show'. All these monologues, as it's called there, sarcastically interpret Trump's handling of the pandemic. The biggest punch of their jokes was Trump's claim in a press conference that he's been taking hydroxychloroquine for a week as a preventive measure against coronavirus, and Nancy Pelosi calls him morbidly obese in part of her response.

For this paper, I would take one example from each country- 'Lallantop' from India and 'The Daily Social Distancing Show' from USA. Lallantop has a segment 'Duniyadari' that deals with the national and international news. The Daily Show is now called as The Daily Social Distancing show. Both these channels address the viewers about the current pandemic and also about the varied aspects of the pandemic, ranging from the medical to the economic. The two monologuers are Saurabh Dwivedi and Trevor Noah. These are actually two different shows with different but interesting layouts. Duniyadari addresses the world issues in serious and sombre tone while Trevor Noah banks on comedy and satire. Both try to be fairly impartial and have the guts to call a spade a spade but Noah is self-acclaimed anti Trump. So, at times, his caricatures go a little far. But both are working incessantly to educate people about what's happening in the world with the pandemic and both dig deep into the raison d'etre of the policies framed by their respective governments regarding the corona virus. Both seek to infuse a ray of hope in the pandemic ridden people in their respective countries, though Dwivedi's range is a tad wider. Noah keeps informing people of the philanthropic works done by the volunteers. For example, Taraji P Henson provides free sessions of virtual therapy to people struggling with the effects of the COVID-19 through her foundation. To quote her, "My prayer and my hope is that people who have shunned seeking help, or believed the stigma around therapy, can take this time and this moment to experience it, to just try it. Because we keep saying, 'when the world opens back up', we will all have trauma to get over after this." And we really need to keep our sanity intact. One difference between their presentations is that Dwivedi prefers presenting before the people how the things stand and reserves giving his opinion, while Noah does give his viewpoint loud and clear.

And the latest happening that's doing the rounds in American media in the backdrop of coronavirus pandemic is the heinous killing of George Floyd. Governor Gavin Newsom says, "The black community is not responsible for what's happening in this country right now-we are, we are, we are. Our institutions are responsible. We are accountable to this moment. Let's just call that out." The killing of George Floyd has totally upended America. But here again, misinformation about George Floyd protests surges on social media. Hundreds of posts are circulating on Twitter and Facebook saying he is not actually dead. The collision of racial tensions and political polarisation during the coronavirus pandemic has supersized the misinformation, researchers say. To quote, "Much of it is being shared by the conspiracy group QAnon and far-right commentators as well as by those on the left." Media is still severed between protecting the rights of the police and being a trailblazer to Black Lives Matter.

An impartial and positive media can definitely come up to heal the world at this moment. It has immense power to manoeuvre public opinion to the creative and compassionate side. Political discussions can be based on facts only if government, opposition and political parties are transparent in their functions otherwise all will be based on rumours and allegations only. Similarly only an educated society and a society aware of its rights can challenge and question the information, misinformation, integration or disintegration, and can identify humanisation or dehumanisation to form a constructive opinion and change. So, it can certainly be reckoned a phase when a big change is round the corner. And with the development of society in terms of enlightenment and a broader vision, people will clearly differentiate between Information and Advertisement which media offers to the viewers.

Note

This paper is based on heavy inputs from Comedy Central UK and Instagram accounts of The Daily Show with Trevor Naoh, The New York Times, The Economic Times, Pew Research Centre, Journalism and Media, and interviews with friends.

13

Exodus of Migrants in Times of Covid-19: An Afterthought

— *Dr. Achla Sonker*

Along routes from Delhi, Mumbai and Gujrat to Uttar Pradesh, Bihar and Orissa migrant workers with their families, children of all age groups, old supported by their sticks and limping, young men and women drenched in sweat bravely facing the fierce sun, on hot and dusty roads carrying heavy bags strapped to their backs, sacks on their heads, holding the babies and young children in their arms, driven by desperation with little food and few bottles of water were walking to their home miles and miles away. This pitiful situation may remind one of the times of partition. Fallen out of cash, jobs and homes ever since a nation-wide lockdown was announced starting March 25, 2020 migrant workers from across the country began to walk and cycle back to their home states. Lockdown due to COVID-19, "has been like a death sentence for the underprivileged,"[1] reflected the economist Jean Dereze, on News 18. Hundreds of thousands of migrant workers, displaced both physically and emotionally, are living in abject penury and on the brink of starvation as the means of their livelihood has stopped. Having a little to hope for and forced by the question of survival, 45 million migrant workers with no choice left with them but to come out on streets; in their determination to walk home they made themselves heard.

There are hordes of people who are part of our daily existence to make our routine chaos manageable from domestic help to drivers, masons, carpenters, painters blended into the landscape from the vegetable sellers to the roadside food stall or *kirana* store boys and still there are some more carrying their trade on their heads and shoulders from *bhel puri* to cobblers or hairdressers. They return home their daily wages earned; in the evening we don't see them either. Yet there are millions of them. "Migrant workers are like nowhere people. Yet, they are everywhere. From high-rises to highway, who builds them? It is a silent army of migrant workers, working day and night with no job security, no social safety net and poor living conditions- yet theirs are not the names we see on the billboards or the foundation stones of these shining symbols of India's economic progress."[2] Migrant workers have long remained invisible to policy and politics, have since ages been taken for granted. But this year's Labour Day had a different message for the whole world to see and realize, "the policies made to contain the pandemic have been made or influenced by a class of people who pay little or no attention to the consequences for the underprivileged."[3] Government has come under fire and faced criticism for overlooking the plight of migrants who have been worst hit by the lockdown.

Stranded workers dismissed by employers, enjoying no protection from the governments, thrown out of their accommodation, and their small savings drying up felt left in the lurch amidst the grave adversity. Distress among unemployed workers kept rising as it became difficult for them to sustain. With trains, buses and public conveyance under locks and gates closed, millions of migrants in an effort to reach back their homes moved out on streets trudging across hundreds of kilometers – some even losing their lives in the attempt. Public Interest Litigation moved before the supreme court seeking compensation for the families of persons, including migrant workers, who have died or injured while walking on roads in an attempt to reach their home states amid COVID-19 clearly brings out the discrimination between interstate workers and migrants in other countries under, 'Vande Bharat' mission by central government to bring back those who were stranded in other countries amid pandemic. "How is that we ran special flights for middle and upper middle class Indians from across the world, but we forgot to organize buses for our poor?"[4] This clearly indicates that the policy makers could have never visualized the extent of the issue of migrant workers as a group big enough to be taken seriously. Now under limelight, governments, policy makers, economists and others know they cannot take migrants lightly.

"Send us home," is the only demand of the migrants. After lot of hue and cry, special packages and relief was announced for the migrants but the sad part of the story is like all the other schemes this too has not been fully able to reach the people for whom it was meant. One of the 200 workers on a construction site in Delhi, Fazulu told a sad story of being handed over hundred rupees each and few kilos of dry ration when the lockdown was first announced and since then they have received nothing. The fear can be seen on their faces, "if something happens to us here, we fall ill from coronavirus or any other disease who will look after us?"[5] Misare, one of 48 construction workers from Madhya Pradesh now living at a wedding venue on the outskirts of Hyderabad in a camp said, "The five hundred rupees promised by authorities (central government) has not been given. We were given 5kg of rice and a kilo of *dal* last month."[6] In Jharkhand a large number of migrants have not received one thousand rupees promised by the state government. Vikash Kumar Singh, 28 year old worker from Karnataka said, "We slept on an empty stomach for several nights, registered on Jharkhand Chief Minister's special assistance scheme app. But I have not received any money till date."[7] The plight is the same for thousands of labours in camps across the country, who are yearning to go back to their villages.

Incidents of stranded migrant workers turning violent in Surat, torching of vegetable carts, damaging vehicles or pelting stones on police in Bengaluru or clashes in Bhagpat border in U.P. reflect upon the anger of migrants of the false promises, lack of assistance and proper arrangements for the migrants. On March 30, over 90 migrant laboures were arrested in Surat for protesting against being barred from returning home. Bansidhar Lenaka, General Secretary of Jagganathpuri charitable trust, which looks into the issues of migrant workers in the industrial city, said, "there are around 25,000 people, just from Orissa, who are working in the embroidery units and textile factory ......since lockdown half of the workers have not got their salaries."[8] Pending wages, no work, demands of the rent by the landlords, lockdown, and extension of it, not able to return to their home or family have left the migrant workers with few options. Naushad Sheikh, a daily wage worker in Ghaziabad who has walked from Delhi to Lucknow 280 km is not the only one. "We saw many laboures returning home," said Shyam Gautam 24, a mason, returning to Sultanpur with Sheikh, "Many more will do the same. We can't survive in cities anymore."[9]

Responding to the demands from migrant workers, and states, the central Government on 1st May allowed special trains to enable the movement of migrants to their home states. 300 Shramik Special trains from Indian railways were to run each day to ferry the stranded migrant workers. National Migrant Information System (NMIS), an online dashboard for the states was put up to record figures so that movement of the people can be monitored. Buses and trucks also were plied along the camps and isolation centers so that the spread of the virus can be checked. With the majority of 10 million migrant workers heading back to Bihar, Uttar Pradesh, Odisha, West Bengal, Jharkhand and Madhya Pradesh, states geared up to receive the migrants. On their return the migrants were to be lodged in quarantine facilities in their native districts for 14 days as states feared that with the migrants the virus can spread rapidly. Odisha chief minister Naveen Patnaik ordered the health department to increase the state capacity to conduct Covid-19 tests by more than four folds, Bihar decided to conduct pool testing of its returning workers, Chief Minister Yogi Adityanath has directed the districts to get medical checkup, testing of the migrants done. Almost all the states were to arrange for the food, shelter and ensure that migrant workers did not face any problems in the quarantine facilities. After the stipulated quarantine the migrants were to be sent home with a ration kit and one thousand rupees each as a sustenance allowance, however migrants have a different story to tell as many of them were caught trying to escape these centers.

There were reports of 25 migrant workers running away from the government run quarantine center in Katihar district because the facilities were inadequate. In government schools and village council buildings thousands of shelters have been set up but many of them lack basic facilities. Many who tried to escape these centers complained of overcrowding, not given any food, filthy toilets, mosquitoes, no electricity or some even having no beds. In the states of Bihar and Uttar Pradesh reports of violation of quarantine by the migrants put a serious question to the administrative authority of these state. "For hundreds of migrant workers who braved hunger and blistered feet to walk, their hardships are far from over as many are facing social boycott or have been denied entry to their villages. Residents of a village in Bengal's Purulia district who returned from Chennai where they worked as labourers had to quarantine themselves on tree branches, tying cloth to make some sort of sitting arrangement."[10] It's not just financial issues but social exclusion too that these migrant have to face. "We reached helpless and hungry, but we were not even allowed to be in our own homes, where do we go? Asked Sajjan Thakur a resident of Rampatti village in Madhubani district, who returned from Noida."[11] At a time when thousands of migrants are returning and state governments are grappling with the herculean task of their isolation, migrants on run could possibly be carriers of coronavirus infection and can pose a serious threat for the people.

The government as a measure to address the problem of migrants not only announced 20 trillion package to revive the Indian economy but also offered free food grains (nationwide usage of Public Distribution System, ration card) and affordable housing (under Pradhan Mantri Awas Yojana) to migrant workers who have been stranded in cities without jobs or money to sustain themselves during lockdown. This is expected to benefit 80 million migrant workers and will cost the center 3,500 crore. A credit facility of 5,000 crore for street vendors was also implemented with a hope that this may encourage poor migrants to stay in cities. The COVID-19 pandemic has hit India's poor the hardest. Finance Minister Nirmala Sitharaman says that 146.2 million person days of work will be generated under MGNREGS with the migrants in mind. There are other plans too in the offing.

Labour Laws

India has a vast number of labour laws, counting 44 which makes labour rights more complicated rather than simplifying it. The process of clubbing them into 4 Labour Codes to make them more comprehensive is underway. The interstate migrant rights are defined in 'The Inter-State Migrant Workmen (Regulation of Employment and Conditions of Service) Act, 1979'. This law requires contractors to get a license from the state from where they intend to bring the labours, thereafter within 15 days they are supposed to provide all details of the labours to the Registering authority with which their establishment is registered. It may be the central or the state government. Contractors are to maintain registers for all migrant workers and provide them a passbook containing details of their employment. The establishment has to provide a displacement allowance of 50% of the wages during any disruption period, along with accommodation and health facilities. The violation may attract jail term of upto a year and a fine of Rs. 1000. Despite it, according to state labour bureaus, less than 5% of the migrant workers are enrolled with government agencies. There is also no provision for companies to file annual reports on migrant workers and allowances paid to them.[12]

The hardships generated due to economic shutdown have brought the migrant labours to the brink. However, some state governments in the name of expediting economic recovery and increasing ease of business, have passed ordinances to modify or suspend labour laws. Uttar Pradesh suspended key labour laws for three years on May 06 through an ordinance. Madhya Pradesh announced on May 7 that it was taking a similar course to put all labour laws on hold, barring some provisions of the Factories Act, 1948, for the next 1000 days.[13] The decision was protested against by the Trade Unions stating that these changes violate workers' rights and are in contravention to ILO Convention No. 144 which India is a signatory to. It necessitates tripartite consultation between the government, employers and the workers. The Central government has asked the state governments not to change these laws in a manner that violates India's commitment to the International Conventions. Though labour laws fall under the concurrent list in the constitution which gives state government also the power to modify them but they need to be ratified at the central level. "Freezing of labour laws can be done for three months, not three years. The main concern is violation of accepted universal norms. Industrial dispute resolution mechanisms, compensation etc. are important considerations. Can you simply suspend all labour laws?" asked an officer of the Union Labour Ministry.[14]

The Centre introduced the Occupational Safety, Health and Working Conditions Code in Lok Sabha in July 2019 to subsume and replace 13 labour laws including the Inter-state Migrant Workmen Act. The Code retains some provisions of the law like contractors having to obtain licenses, the displacement and journey allowances, but the penal provision has been excluded. A Parliamentary panel has recommended a separate chapter on migrant workers in the code and said that every state should have a helpline for them like the Odisha government along with seasonal hostels for them and their children, as well as strengthening anti-human trafficking units and the setting up of migration support centres. The Labour Ministry plans to accept the recommendations.[15]

Steps Underway

Returning migrant workers provide an opportunity to reshape state's economic ecosystem. Though it will be challenging to provide jobs to all of them, the planning and efforts for that need to be started and undertaken in all earnest. Uttar Pradesh government has formed a Migration Commission to prepare a data base of all returning migrants and do skill mapping through district level employment exchanges. They will be given apprenticeship as per their skills and the state government intends to generate 20 lakh employment opportunities for migrant workers[16] by attracting investments in the state by the companies exiting China in the wake of Covid-19, and other channels.

To resolve the problem faced in drawing ration in states other than the origin state, the central government has approved the 'One Nation, One Ration Card' scheme. As on June 18th, 2020, 20 states have already joined it while others are expected to come overboard. The centre plans to implement the facility fully across the country by March 2021, under which eligible beneficiaries would be able to avail their entitled food grains under the National Food Security Act (NFSA) from any fair price shop in the country using the same ration card.[17]

Parliamentary Standing Committee on Labour is pushing for a portable social security number for migrant workers and other employees in the vast unorganized sector. The unique social security number, which would be linked to the Aadhaar unique identity number, is expected to automatically identify unorganized sector workers and help the government roll out targeted doles or welfare schemes for them in a more organized way.[18]

Conclusion

Migrant workers form the backbone of the economic system in a country like India, with a huge number of 65 million inter-state migrants out of which 33% are workers as per the Census 2011.[19] Failure to provide the security, adequate food, and cash relief to the hasty attempts at responding to industry demands to hold labours captive and pushing ill-conceived labour reforms has exposed deep faults in the policy making of the government. The lockdown made visible the indignities migrant workers suffer but it also served as a reminder of how effectively workers can protest against the state. Workers voted with their feet choosing long arduous journey home rather than to face the uncertainties of inhospitable cities. But the question is when there is time to kick-start the economies on the track again, we will need them. We have underestimated the role migrants played in the economy. We have failed to recognize their contribution. We knew they existed but never acknowledged their strength. This is a time when we should rethink, revise and restart to build laws to protect rights and restore dignity of the workers. Can one imagine smart and big cities like Mumbai, Hyderabad, Gujrat or Chennai without migrant worker? You can reopen industries, but one must think who runs them? The pandemic has provided an opportunity to initiate and complete a long-pending task- to rebuild an economic system based on ethical values of labour, an inclusive and equitable system which makes these foundational stones an equal participant in the fruits of their labour. The time is now to harness their latest strength in a more humane and organized way.

References

1. Tully, Mark; 'India's Migrant workers.......', Sunday Hindustan Times, Lucknow, 10 May, 2020, p. 8.
2. Ghatak, Maitreesh; 'The indispensability of labour in reviving India's economic engine,' Hindustan Times, Lucknow, 9 May, 2020, p. 8.
3. Tully, Mark; 'India's Migrant workers deserve better than this', Sunday Hindustan Times, Lucknow, 10 May, 2020, p. 8.
4. Dutt, Barkha; 'Migrant workers are being treated poorly. Address their concern, now,' Hindustan Times, Lucknow, 18 April, 2020, p. 8.
5. Dutt Barkha, 'Migrant workers are being treated poorly. Address their concern, now,' Hindustan Times, Lucknow, 18 April, 2020, p. 8.
6. Hindustan Times, Lucknow, 18 April, 2020, p. 5.
7. Hindustan Times, Lucknow, 6 May, 2020, p. 6.
8. Sunday Hindustan Times, Lucknow, 12 April, 2020, p. 7.
9. Hindustan Times, Lucknow, 18 April, 2020, p. 5.
10. http://www.timesofindia.indiatimes.com, 27 May 2020, 16:30.
11. http://www.timesofindia.indiatimes.com, 27 May 2020, 16:30.
12. Chauhan Chetan, 'Migrant workers law in focus as crisis intensifies', Hindustan Times, Lucknow, May 29, 2020, p. 10.
13. Haq Zia, 'States labour law changes under central govt scanner', Hindustan Times, Lucknow, June 01, 2020, p. 4.
14. Haq Zia, 'States labour law changes under central govt scanner', Hindustan Times, Lucknow, June 01, 2020, p. 4.
15. Chauhan Chetan, 'Migrant workers law in focus as crisis intensifies', Hindustan Times, Lucknow, May 29, 2020, p. 10.
16. Varma Gyan, Anuja, 'Migrant database: Job exchanges push UP's massive skill-mapping exercise', Livemint, Updated: 26 May 2020, 10:48 AM IST, https://www.livemint.com/news/india/migrant-database-job-exchanges-push-up-s-massive-skill-mapping-exercise-11590468094916.html
17. 'One Nation, One Ration Card scheme/ Ram Vilas Paswan to approach Telecom Minister regarding Internet problem in hilly areas', The Hindu, updated June 18, 2020, 18:19 IST, https://www.thehindu.com/news/national/one-nation-one-ration-card-ram-vilas-paswan-to-approach-telecom-minister-regarding-internet-problem-in-hilly-states/article31861683.ece
18. Chatterji Saubhadra, 'Social security ID for migrants on top of labour panel's agenda', Hindustan Times, Updated: Jun 03, 2020 05:59 IST, New Delhi, https://www.hindustantimes.com/india-news/social-security-id-for-migrants-on-top-of-labour-panel-s-agenda/story-YwyFjHQgrorT0bxKB1qIlI.html

19. Singh Sushant, 'Explained: Indian Migrants across India', The Indian Express, New Delhi, Updated: April 29, 2020 8:03:50 pm, https://indianexpress.com/article/explained/coronavirus-india-lockdown-migran-workers-mass-exodus-6348834/#:~:text=His%20estimates%2C%20which%20are%20based,of%20these%20migrants%20are%20workers.

14

Impact of COVID-19 on Politics

— *Colonel Kuldip Singh Grewal (Retd)*

In December 2019 when Covid -19, a highly infectious disease caused by a novel Corona virus (SARS COV-2) was spreading through the population in Wuhan and causing devastation, politicians all over the world were engaged in playing political games in their respective countries absolutely unaware of the viral fury that was waiting to engulf their people. China was trying hard to subdue the viral invasion which had already turned lethal. The World Health Organization though aware of the situation failed to highlight the danger to the world and caution other nations. Then on 10 January WHO woke up from its slumber and issued a warning about the spread of the Novel Corona; the advisory was to detect, test and manage potential cases based on what was known about the virus at that time. The first case of Covid-19 outside China was reported from Thailand on 13 January 2020. China though carried on with its regular flights to other countries till some cases of viral infection surfaced in Italy followed by other countries.

The WHO could not make up its mind about the level of threat of this new Corona virus even after a joint mission to China had submitted its report on 24 February highlighting the seriousness and dangers of the new Corona Virus. It was not declared as a pandemic till 11 March 2020. Meanwhile India was busy in organizing a political exercise for the arrival of Donald Trump, the grand "Namaste Trump" extravaganza and the handling of the Delhi riots almost simultaneously. Meanwhile the danger of the novel Corona Virus was growing ever more acute but the political bandwidth was further occupied in the overturn of the state government of Madhya Pradesh.

Factors Affecting Political Shift

It is people of the country especially in democracies who decide about the body of politicians suitable to steer the country as per their aspirations. The average age of the population, Education, Economic conditions, Demography, Religion, Culture and Traditions are major factors which influence the formation of political bodies to run the country. Fast paced development and interdependence among countries of the world has grown significantly. The relationship with other nations depends on a country's own interests in defence, trade, economic gains, cultural and ethnic similarities, geographical proximity and political accessibility.

Changing Global Politics

"A public health emergency, combined with a global recession has the potential to change politics around the world."[1]

By the end of March 2020 Covid-19 had caused devastation throughout the world, sparing no country from the developed world in Europe and USA to far flung Asian and African countries. France, Kazakhstan, Nigeria, Kenya, Uganda, Ghana and other African countries summoned Chinese ambassadors to question the delays and misinformation provided by China about the origin and spread of the Novel Corona Virus. Instead of accepting their mistakes the Chinese reacted with threats and warnings. The Netherland was asked to behave otherwise China threatened to withhold medical aid supplied by it.

China being the major supplier of Personal Protective Equipment (PPE), Testing Kits and N-95 Masks enhanced its business by supplying such material. A lot of the testing equipment proved unreliable and the PPE proved to be defective. Many countries returned the same. The Chinese Government got away by blaming one of its companies which supplied such equipment, but consignees exposed it as a fraud played on them. Germany demanded $ 160 billion from China for damages caused by the Virus which erupted from Wuhan, spread of which Chinese kept under wraps till it knocked on the doors of those countries that had crucial trade ties with them.

When USA started feeling unbearable pain of rising deaths due to Covid-19, President Donald Trump squarely blamed China for this pandemic and demanded $ 10 million for every American's death. As the US President's election is scheduled on 03 November 2020 Trump's worries are compounding with every US citizen's death due to Covid-19. Hundreds of US companies had moved to China bringing with them the latest technology and in 2017 the US had $336 billion trade deficit with China. USA is China's major trading partner. As Covid-19 is playing havoc in USA with death toll nearing one lakh the mistrust has grown to such an extent that US demanded inquiry into the origin of virus and Australia has also joined in this rhetoric. World over a backlash is building against China for its casual attitude towards the impending calamity. When France also joined the chorus against China over human neglect paving way for Corona Tsunami, China reacted sharply that French left old people to die in their Nursing Homes. Hapless Trump said, "It came from China. We are not happy about it. We just signed a trade deal, the ink wasn't dry and all of a sudden this floated in. We are not going to take it lightly."[2] Many countries expressed similar views and China landed in precarious situation of being isolated. In world politics China slipped to the edge.

Chinese React

Trump led a campaign against its most preferred trade partner to push the Chinese to the wall, but China took the campaigners head on by moving their army of diplomats to blunt the tirade. They issued warnings to small nations to fall in line and keep away from its criticism. China has tried to divert the attention of the world from its purported dubious role in spreading Corona virus by deploying maritime might in South China Sea and Indian Ocean thus forcing USA to sail its warships to disputed areas. Chinese army intrusion in Sikkim's Naku La pass area where in the face off with Indian troops some soldiers were injured was part of diversionary tactics used for warding off corona campaign against it. Also, China enhanced its troops in Ladakh. It intruded in Galwan valley, Demchok and Pangong lake and a stand-off ensued between India and China. The Chinese troops have "come in" about 3 km into Indian territory South East of the Galwan Valley, largely known as Hot Springs area in eastern Ladakh. Beijing has also moved in men at the "finger areas" of Pangong Lake while increasing build up on its side of the Line of Actual Control (LAC).[3]

Simultaneously China instigated Nepal to rake up the Kalapani-Lipulekh issue with India by releasing a new map showing both as its own territory. In addition, China passed a new Security Law for Hong Kong that undermines the autonomy provided to Hong Kong under the Basic Law. With this, China will be entitled to make security laws for Hong Kong, a right which was reserved for the Hong Kong Legislative Council till now. China got embroiled with Vietnam too as Chinese ship entered Vietnamese EEZ (Exclusive Economic Zone) in South China Sea. All these moves are viewed by experts as China's attempts to divert the world's attention from its alleged role in Covid-19 origin and spread, as well as to raise the nationalism plank to assuage the domestic population which shows the signs of discontentment on the authorities' handling of the disease.

Role of the World Health Organisation

World Health Organisation (WHO) was established on 7 April 1948. This day is also celebrated as World Health Day. Dr. Tedros Adhanom Ghebreyesus an Ethiopian citizen is an elected Director General of WHO. It is believed that China canvassed vigorously for Tedros' election in 2017- the first non-practicing physician to hold this Post. Many countries especially where the Covid-19 effect is devastating accuse WHO of concealing the facts of origin and spread of this Novel corona virus. They demand a fair probe as to how it developed into a pandemic. As the voice for a transparent inquiry became louder, WHO agreed to conduct a fair probe. China reacted sharply to this. It is a fact that WHO took extraordinarily high time to warn the world of the impending disaster. It is still not clear whether WHO's snail paced move was by omission or commission to cover up China's negligence. Also it did not issue any advisory to China to stop outgoing flights so as to contain the virus in Wuhan itself. USA, accusing China of overshadowing the working of WHO snapped ties with this organisation.

Impact on Indian Politics

The first general election in India was held from 25 October 1951 to 21 February 1952 after India became independent on 15 August 1947. The Congress Party came into power by winning 364 seats out of a total of 489. Jawahar Lal Nehru became the first Prime Minister of India. Since then the Congress Party ruled the country for most of the time barring few stints by other parties but for the last six years the NDA led by BJP is ruling the country with a clear majority in the Lok Sabha. Of late politics in India has started revolving around religion. Divisive politics has taken root in the world's biggest democracy. The Government of India had come to know about the ferocity and speed of spread of Covid-19 by 21 Feb 2020 when Italy had imposed a partial lockdown. However, the government focus was kept on pushing the NRC and CAA. The protests against NRC and CAA were given communal colour by not only Muslim leaders but also by the ruling dispensation loudmouths. It was the politicians who ignited the communal riots in Delhi which resulted in huge loss of life and property. The Prime Minister stated on April 14 during his address, "Long before we had even single case of Covid-19, India had started screening travellers coming in from Covid-19 affected countries"[4] but this claim is being contested by many in political circles. In fact, only thermal screening was done that too for a few countries' passengers and all the International Airports were not covered. Infected people who had not developed symptoms kept pouring in. Since Nepal border was porous, some Covid-19 affected people may have entered through that. By this time Corona had not only sounded its entry through incoming flights at all 34 International Airports from most affected countries but also alerted the government to start inward testing and apply the concept of home quarantine. The onset of any calamity unifies the nation; the reaction of the people during *Janta* curfew justifies this statement.

Justification of Lockdown

"Lockdown will damage life more than deaths due to Corona Virus."[5] Lockdowns are regarded as cover up to initial failures in violation of "Nip the problem in the bud". Having gauged the people's response to *Janta* Curfew on 22 March, PM Modi ordered nationwide lockdown for 21 days restricting the movement of 1.3 billion people. The people of India were not prepared for this long lockdown as there was hardly any time given to them to reach their destinations, or collect stock of daily needs for three weeks. State governments were asked to arrange for essential supplies to the needy, but they failed due to lack of resources and unpreparedness. As all big and small industries were shut, construction work had come to a standstill, daily wagers and contract employees were rendered jobless without any secured income. Industrialists, and Contractors raised their hands and declared helplessness in their ability to help the workers financially. Most of the daily wagers (mostly migrants) lived in congested areas in shared accommodation. The Media was abuzz with news of deadly virus with specific character of human to human transmission and no cure was visible in near future. The government advised the people to maintain physical distance to save themselves from contacting the viral disease. With nothing to eat and with no money in hand, the overcrowded dwellings combined with media's hysterical reporting of the news caused fear psychosis among hapless migrants and they decided to leave their hovels and came out on the roads. Since there was no transport available, they took the journey on foot to their villages without food, water or even shoes. Politicians retreated to safe places, governments failed to check the migrants' exodus and these poor souls were left to their fate. They endured hunger, governments' apathy, police atrocities and vagaries of weather. Many of them were killed in accidents while travelling in non-passenger vehicles or sleeping on railway tracks and many others died of hunger and diseases.

Politics over Exodus

Congress President Sonia Gandhi declared that State Congress units will pay for the conveyance of migrants who are walking to their destination. The BJP reacted fearing loss of face in case opposition parties undertake this service and requested the government to run Shramik Trains. After getting permission from the Uttar Pradesh Chief Minister, Congress placed around 800 buses at the disposal of U.P. government who however returned the same due to some observations. In the whole scenario "Corona" may not have impacted politics that much but the exodus of migrants will have a lasting effect which will be visible in coming states elections.

Impact on Elections

Covid-19 has disrupted the schedules of election in many countries like general elections in Ethiopia, Iran, Serbia and primary US Presidential election while India has already postponed its Rajya Sabha election which was due on 26 March 2020. Sri Lanka might conduct elections in June 2020 whereas Russia, Italy and United Kingdom where regional assembly, local bodies and regional elections are due may also have to change the dates.[6]

As is expected the Corona virus is here to stay till a vaccine is developed. It is not likely in near future so will the countries carry on with the present governments? No, Some ways and means will have to be found out to conduct regular election which is the soul of democracy. Advanced countries are competent to develop digitalized and incorruptible election system but in India we do not have even updated list of voters and most of the electorates are illiterate. In our country where even EVMs are under scrutiny there is an uncertainty and doubt of a new complex digital system in the minds of the voters in general. The acceptance of such an idea will take time.

Most of the prospective candidates for elections are spending sleepless nights as in the prevailing environment they will not be able to hire demonstrators for the traditional rallies for a show of strength to sway the voters in their favour. Though canvassing through social media, television debates, print media will become potent handles but only for those who can afford the financial burdens of such luxuries. Poor candidates will be hard placed to find a space in open canvassing. Introduction of a government paid election channel wherein all candidates including independents get equal time to convey their views to the public may be a viable answer.

Solutions

Politics deals with everything which aims at smooth running of government of a country or an area. Good politics means good governance. The people at helm of affairs are elected, selected, nominated or appointed to run the affair by executable planning activities dealing with development of the area under their governance. Honesty and character being important personal attributes need to be inherent in a potential politician. Criminals should have no place in politics. Generally it is believed that politicians breed on falsehood. Some politicians being illiterate or semi-literate and clueless of their job play in the hands of bureaucrats. Corrupt people should have no place in the government. Professionals should be preferred with pre- fixed educational qualifications so as to run the government in right direction. Accountability should be central in political set-up. Transparency in all deals will enhance trust of the people in the government. While dealing with invasion of Covid-19 some omissions on the part of top political leaders were quite glaring. They lacked foresightedness, planning and ability to take quick decisions. Therefore there is a need to introduce a system wherein all prospective candidates for election will be required to pass a test which would assess their basic intelligence, ability to plan and decision making. Such tests can be conducted by an autonomous body. To weed out criminals Election Commission should be vested with more powers to deal with rogue politicians and rule-breaking political parties.

Civil Society Initiatives

Civil society organisations play a very important role in shaping the policies of a nation and contributing to the world politics. Due to digital media people are more aware now and express their view points more openly. In today's time, geopolitics is closely interrelated with economics. As nations after nations suffered with the onslaught of Covid-19 and suspicion on China grew, the discontent spread in the citizens, and people have been vocal against the Chinese. A campaign has been initiated against the Chinese goods to attack on the root of the Dragon's power-its trade in cheap goods. The video by noted environmentalist from Ladakh Mr. Sonam Wangchuck which is being widely circulated on social media is a live example of it, in which he exhorts people to answer the Chinese with their wallet power by boycotting its products.[7]

Conclusion

The United States had put all its eggs in the Chinese basket thus making its supposed enemy No.1 into a giant manufacturing hub which supplies all types of goods to most of the countries of the world including Europe and USA. During the Covid-19 breakout, China supplied Personal Protective Kits, Respirators, Test Kits, Ventilators and Masks to Iran, Serbia, USA, Italy and most of African countries thus bursting the myth of US and European superiority. Some countries including India reported that Chinese goods were defective and lacked efficacy. Side effects of Covid-19 might cause political shake ups, toppling of governments, change in system of governments and slashing human rights in some countries. Democracies are more vulnerable to political upheavals than autocracies.

Some countries including the US threatened to call back its companies from China to which India feels a sense of inflated importance that major chunk of those units might land in its lap but the complexity of US-China trade may not let it happen. With the Corona virus effect India may have to look inwards and use indigenous innovation and talent to develop a manufacturing base. Leaders will have to take into consideration the local hardships faced by people, understand their aspirations and provide a vision to rebuild and remould the entire economic ecosystem based largely on self-sufficiency. This shifting inwards will also impact the international relationships. The wave against globalisation which was already underway before the pandemic, has suddenly acquired enormous force. The world will have to create new systems to engage with each other with reduced trade and less physical contact due to the fear. The major challenge in front of the world politics will be to unite against the expansionist and deceitful regime and usher in a new world system based on mutual understanding and cooperation.

References

1. Rachman, Gideon, Financial Times, 28 Feb 2020, 7.20 PM.
2. Rohatgi, Anubha from Washington, Press Trust of India, 29 May 2020.

3. https://theprint.in/defence/chinese-troops-challenge-india-at-multiple-locations-in-eastern-ladakh-standoff-continues/428304/, Philip Alex Snehesh, Chinese troops challenge India at multiple locations in eastern Ladakh, standoff continues, The Print, 24 May 2020, 1.36 pm IST.
4. PMO Ind, 15 March 2020, posted by Wire Staff, 15 April 2020.
5. Prof. Levitt, Micheal, Novel Prize Laureate in Chemistry 2013, telegraph.co.uk, 23 May 2020 8.30 pm.
6. https://economictimes.indiatimes.com/news/international/world-news/covid-19-makes-a-mess-of-election-schedules-around-the-world/articleshow/75416027.cms?from=mdr, Vishnoi Anubhuti, Covid-19 makes a mess of elections around the world, The Economic Times, April 27, 2020, 11.50 pm, IST.
7. https://www.youtube.com/watch?v=MmN-bYho9sY, Stop China Taking Ladakh from India, June 8, 2020, 7.20 pm.

Index

C

G

H

I

N

U

V

W

Y

Z